A Shield for the Columbia River

The Quarantine Station and the U.S. Public Health Service at Knappton Cove, WA and Astoria, OR

1890-1899

Friedrich E. Schuler

A Shield for the Columbia River: The Quarantine Station and the U.S. Public
Health Service at Knappton Cove, WA and Astoria, OR 1890-1899

Designed by Andrea Janda

For Mav

Nancy Anderson has the first and last word when it comes to Knappton Cove Quarantine Station. Everything we know we know from her and the group of enthusiasts she gathers. I, an immigrant to our country, had the privilege of joining them for which I am deeply grateful.

These pages are a simple attempt to add a few additional stories to her existing ones. This book is a humble addition to what we know already. Thus, at best, it is a partial interpretation. For the next generation of historians much history remains to be added.

Key to improved understanding will be the realization that events in Astoria and Knappton took place next to what happened in Port Townsend, Tacoma, Washington D.C., and Angel Island, California. There would not exist a station at Knappton Cove without the events taking place at these other west coast locations but also across the Pacific Ocean, the Panama Canal even the Atlantic Ocean. It was never just a Columbia River story.

This book is not the final word about what happened at the station. At its center merely stand stories based on the rediscovered primary sources of the station now located at the National Archives in Washington, D.C. No doubt, other scholars will find other new collections and should correct what is being argued on the following pages.

In these pages the story of the station is about the unique historical situation around the mouth of the Columbia between 1894 and 1900. Astoria and the Washington side of Columbia River were a unique American place often, unfortunately, still isolated from national consideration. Events taking place in Astoria are never stereotypical of anything.

The text is also about the U.S. Public Health Service, then called the U.S. Marine Hospital Service. Its service men and women used science and neutral verified data coming from abroad to protect this bay against other smaller priorities lacking a bird's eye perspective or the willingness to consider the larger world. That some used the situation to settle racist scores confirms that it is typical of our ongoing historical experiment to build a better more equal United States of America.

So much in our country is so frequently contested and all voices want to be not just heard but also want to be winners. Then Life itself teaches that, ultimately, it is about something different than being successful. Life giving deep human bonds remain the top prize, not being number one.

A special thank you to Nancy's daughter Heather, Nancy's entire family, the board members of Knappton Cove Heritage Center and retired P.H.S. officer Jay Paulsen for their enthusiasm, friendship and open reception.

At Clatsop County Historical Society I am forever indebted to Liisa Penner and her wonderful help and resources. At the Astoria Library the entire staff and the thoughtful and dedicated library director Jimmy Pearson made the difference. John Goodenberger is an appreciated friend. At the Appello Historical Archive in Naselle Patty and Kelly Shumar repeatedly were gracious and always inspiring.

A thank you to Jeff Smith's support at Astoria's Columbia River Maritime Museum. Finally, Susan Wladaver-Morgan put a shine onto the text.

A special word of appreciation at the colleagues at Portland State University who were patient with my work and left me alone at the right time. These people helped. Especially Tim Garrison and John Ott.

On the layout level Dr. Andrea Janda pulled it all together. Without her the journey from my thoughts to the bookshelf would not have happened the way it did. In addition she always found ways to whisper to the computer when it tried to have a mind of its own. The PSU History Department is so much richer because of her amazing work. And a Liquorice pipe shoutout to Dr. Jeff Brown. Long Live true Historians! The last and most special shoutout to my peeps in Washington and Berlin.

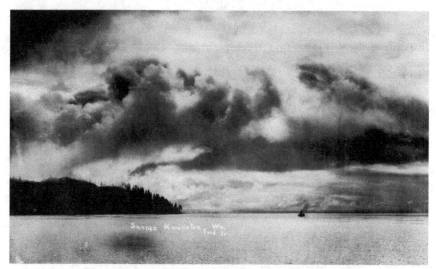

Courtesy Appelo Archive, Naselle, WA; Sunrise view from the Knappton side of the Columbia, before 1900.

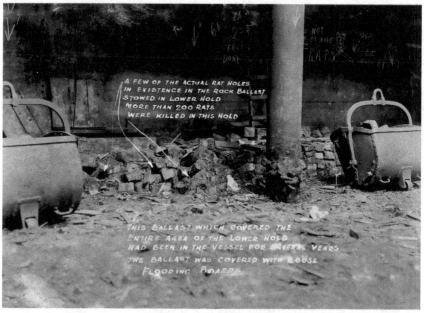

Courtesy National Archive of the United States (hereafter cited as NAUS), RG 90, Educational picture detailing ballast consisting of hay and rocks from lower hold of a vessel, around 1900.

On a dry day, the bay near Knappton stretches gently toward the paddler looking for a place to beach his lead canoe calmly. Chinook and other Native American tribal members traveling by boat, at least on occasion, must have enjoyed a temporary stop at this bend in the river. I know they fished there as well. Such a lodge was a temporary house where ill people were wrapped in steam until their disease was sweated out of them, floating it up into the sky; it was a place supposed to heal both their body and soul.

For Native Americans steam drove away impurities that caused disease and literally steamed illness out of their bodies into the sky. After 1900, at the same bay, western medical practitioners would again enlist steam. There, inside a quarantine station's disinfection building, closed iron steamers would use water vapor to boil and burn viruses and bacteria out of passenger's clothes and suitcases. In addition, sulfur vapor was blown into ships' hulls to counteract any contamination in the ballast that then most often consisted of stones and hay they carried into U.S. territory from lands across the Pacific Ocean.

For native people, building a sweat lodge and heating stones inside it were seen as spiritual processes. Western medicine, by contrast, decided in favor of a bureaucratic process. Neither Native Americans nor European Americans understood that the particles the vapor carried into the sky were not the real carriers of smallpox, cholera, plague, or yellow fever.

The community and its doctors failed again and again to realize that death would float into this U.S. port hiding inside fleas, still clinging to the putrid fur of rats eager to discover America. Again and again they did not identify the correct action that would have stopped the global journey of deadly dangers. Until then, in truth, not much could be done besides keeping up rituals to calm the sense of lostness.

Frightened European Americans tamed their sense of helplessness by embossing prayers on bleached paper chanted by what they called a bureaucrat, as if the plague could be frightened away by paper tattooed with rules and regulations. Late 19th century people insisted on such bureaucratic mantras in hope they would become the building blocks to wall out nature. They assured themselves that such words on paper, reprinted and distributed to official offices, were somehow more effective than the sound of the prayers of medicine men and women. Bureaucratic principles were once again projected across vast geographical territories, including our Northwest. It was the second tool European Americans used to encircle invisible natural foreign agents.

And yet, given what people knew at that time, such a paradox was alright to stomach because doctors kept repeating and repeating their attempt to unlock the truth. Until human efforts across the world found the correct explanation, words and principles were attached to the person everybody was supposed to heed, not just anybody, but a bureaucrat called a health commissioner. He was the third tool to further reduce anxiety about responsibility to destroy the persistently invisible forces of disease. At least one person was now officially in charge of realizing the state's health policy so that citizens could go on with their daily lives. In reality, he too could not stop the plague. Nevertheless, having a single person in charge provided personalized focus for concerned people which was far better than experiencing random outbreaks at unpredictable locations where plague, fevers, and smallpox made a mockery out of print, principles, and politician's assertions.

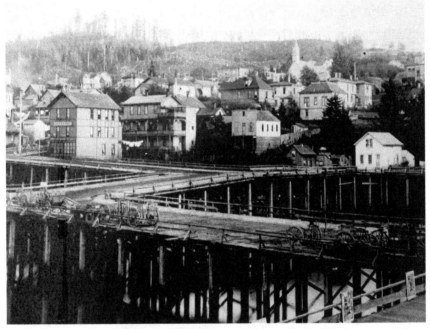

Courtesy Clatsop County Historical Society, Astoria, Oregon, Early Astoria.

Putting one person in charge theoretically promised healthy, measured human direction while ill citizens waded through the fog of war drifting in from the battle for greater health and longer life. The official title "officer of health" promised to elevate the battle from the level of tribe, a form of social organization European Americans officially did not like, to the level of the government of the state of Oregon, which somehow implied effectiveness and service to all citizens. Moreover, the officer was proclaimed to act scientifically. His prescription, therefore, had to be obeyed, regardless of one's prayers or feelings. Thus, a new form of society and culture emerged at the mouth of the Columbia: a "tribe" gathered around science, self-identified as modern, and motivated by long-distance trade across the Pacific.

In the 1870s, the emerging state of Oregon's increasing demands for self-determined local life were published in Bellinger and Cotton's "Annotated Codes and Statutes of Oregon." The volume stated that Oregon's governor would appoint one health officer who had to live in Astoria. Most importantly, he was to investigate every vessel arriving from the Pacific Ocean for contagious diseases, particularly smallpox, cholera, and leprosy.

Overnight our nondescript bay found itself near Oregon's most important town to confront incoming foreign pathogens. If real health-related discoveries were ever to be made, and if paper, principle, and talk could become reliable action this bay would be only six miles away from the center of action.

Astorians reacted with practicality. They designated Smith Point, on the Columbia River at the west end of Astoria, as a place where all things biological, invisible, and dangerous were to be sequestered. There, plague, yellow fever, and beriberi would have to sit on a vessel surrounded by cold water, as if the water formed a moat that kept infection from landing on U.S. soil.

Yet nobody defined who would or could do what if a ship with 100 people dying from the plague were ever to anchor there.

To be fair, minor actions had been spelled out. As ships made it across the Columbia bar, all had to give notice to Astoria's health officer. He was then obliged to make the short trip from downtown to the ship anchored at Smith Point and raise a red flag at its main mast. That meant others had to stop all interaction with the ship until it was declared disinfected. If the health officer found an infected passenger or crew member on board, he was to bring him or her to Astoria to a location of his choice. The cost of this quarantine treatment would be charged to the ship's owner or sometimes the infected person himself.[1] Once the ship was deemed free of dangerous contamination it could raise anchor at Smith Point and either the current would move it back to Astoria's wharf or it could venture on east, up the Columbia, toward Portland.

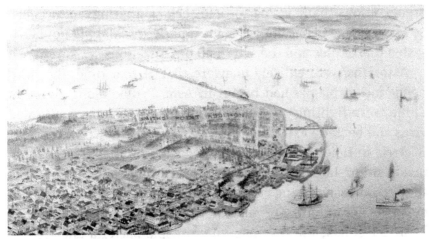

Courtesy Astoria, Oregon, Public Library, Smith Point, Astoria, map 1898.

All these printed words and minor regulations were nothing but a distraction from the ugly truth that in case of plague, everybody would help themselves as they saw fit. They could reasonably be expected to disregard all principles that modern states had proclaimed. Social rules would likely break down completely and fast.

[1] Annotated Codes and Statutes of Oregon, Chapter XIX, of Quarantine of Vessels, Volume 2. L. 1870, P. 101.

For example, in the 1600s, in the Danish fishing town Holm, near Schleswig, (today Germany), the arrival of the plague caused the complete abandonment of all reliable social behavior. The simplest courtesy between neighbors disappeared quickly.[2] This experience of the arrival of plague and the following social chaos was so hurtful that the Danish inhabitants created a written code of how to deal with plague. It detailed who would retrieve a dead body from a home; which neighbor or friend had to attend a funeral; even what people had to wear as they dealt with a dead person. This code led to the creation of mutual self-help organizations that have performed social gatherings until today. So far, the plague has not yet made it back to Schleswig nor has it tested these rules and the self-help organizations.

Astorians were entirely unaware that at that time, the third pandemic of plague had begun in Asia. People along rivers in China were fighting civil wars, and troop movements afforded virus and bacteria extra rapid transport up and down waterways. Bacteria in fluids inside fleas hitched rides on the rats scurrying inside ships' hulls sailing down river toward the Pacific. There they could easily change carriers and scurry onto ships ready to cross the ocean for San Francisco, Seattle, and Astoria.

In the 1880s, the invisible, microscopic bacteria and viruses were endangering Chinese and Indian people but not yet Astorians. Still, infectious organisms from Asia had begun to add an indirect distant threat to Astorians' lives. Those first exposed to the threat were people being brought from Asia to work as contract laborers gutting salmon in Astoria's growing canning industry.

In 1871, George Hume first hired former miners from Southern Oregon to come north and work in his canneries.[3] Scandinavian

---

[2] Germany, Schleswig, City Museum display about hamlet of Holm, 2019.
[3] Nancy Bell Anderson, Heather Bell Henry, ed.; The Columbia River's Ellis Island, The Story of Knappton Cove, (Gearhart: self-published, 2012), p. 36-38.

immigrants were also hired to fish the abundant salmon out of the Columbia. Four years later, 12 canneries between Astoria and Portland depended on contract laborers. When Humes opened the Eureka and Epicure Packing Company in 1876, it was furthest from his mind that he had also opened the building that would one day be used as part of a quarantine station.

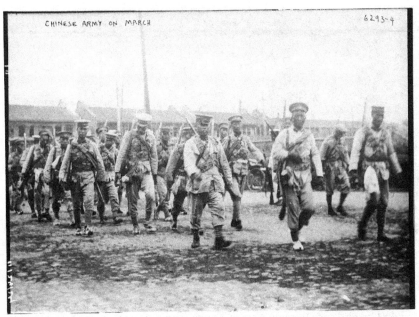

Courtesy U.S. Library of Congress (hereafter cited as LOC), Bains News Service, Chinese army on march, 1900.

There, former Chinese American miners were placed next to recently transported contract laborers from Canton, China.[4] That was the region where the plague was raging. Soon Scandinavians were steering over 1,000 gillnet boats back and forth across the Columbia catching enough fish to keep 30 canneries in operation.

[4] Pacific Fishermen: Year Book, (1920), based on Columbia Riverimages.com/regions/places. Accessed 2018.

Many do not realize that these labor practices had brought a third culture of health to Knappton Cove. After Native American's practicing rituals of health in sweat lodges and European Americans entrusting their future to bureaucracy, Chinese Americans opened their pockets as portable medicine cabinets filled with herbs they had minced and then rolled up into pills.

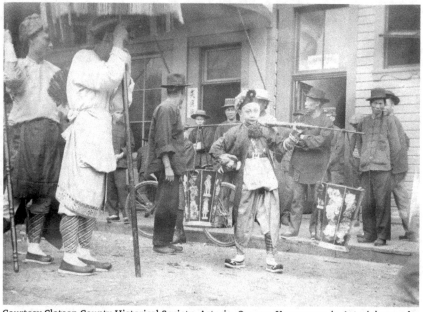

Courtesy Clatsop County Historical Society, Astoria, Oregon, Young man in Astoria's parade wearing his traditional Chinese festival outfit around 1900.

Add a little lint to the mix and you can envision workers medicating themselves inside this large, rectangular, wooden building. In Wahkiakum County, one-third of the total population of 4,000 consisted of men from China.[5] A bitter little pill from their pants pockets might have made bearable the merciless, slimy, and bloody manual labor at Hume's cannery while Finnish

[5] HistoryLink.org, "The first Salmon Cannery on the Columbia River opens at Eagle Cliff, Wahkiakum Country in 1866 by Kit Oldham," Dec 20, 2006; accessed 2/3/2015.

American boat operators again used steam piped into a *sauna* and Finnish-speaking doctors. Suddenly, however, a voice from the U.S. East Coast interfered in Oregon's and Astoria's other cultures of health. By 1878, politicians in Washington, D.C., had decided that the federal government was responsible for dealing with diseases arriving on foreign ships. The newly created national quarantine act of 1878 thus challenged anew regional and local efforts at dealing with health issues arriving on ships from abroad. In addition, there now existed inside the U.S. Treasury a Bureau of Navigation, but since its creation in July of the same year, it had hired only 50 employees nationwide. It could project no presence or power into Astoria's cultures.

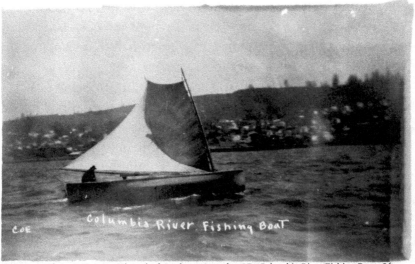

Courtesy Clatsop County Historical Society, Astoria, OR, *Columbia River Fishing Boat. Often immigrants from Finland operated them and worked as fishermen.*

Still, at least in theory, keeping foreign pathogens out of Astoria and from there, up the Columbia, was becoming a competitive affair in which men from the nation's capital rivaled men selected in Salem, Oregon, who also wanted to dominate doctors practicing in Astoria.

On Washington's side on the river, regional politicians repeated the creation of structures that Oregonians had already established across the bay. On October 29, 1881, the legislature in Olympia passed House Bill No. 59. It offered "an act to provide against the spread of infectious contagious disease and in relation to quarantine of vessels in Pacific County." In November, Governor W.A. Newell signed it into law. Four months later, in February 1882, the Board of Health of Washington's Pacific County adopted unified health regulations. Maritime quarantine regulations for Puget Sound were also created and published that month. As in Oregon, the hope for health received an identifiable face: E.T. Balch became Pacific County's health officer.

But what did this really mean? There was still no hospital in Washington's Pacific County. In cases where someone became ill with smallpox or plague, men and women had to be isolated on land in existing or temporary local pest houses.

It would be a significant misunderstanding to believe that a federal quarantine station was supposed to keep smallpox out of the Columbia region. Smallpox was already a regular resident, certainly in Clatsop County, just not in epidemic proportions.

In 1862, a smallpox plague had traveled up the coast from San Francisco to Victoria, B.C. and on to Alaska. In April of that year, it had passed Astoria and continued north, reaping traumatic havoc among Native American communities living around Puget Sound.[6] In 1881, the Astoria Daily Bulletin confirmed that smallpox still endangered all people in town,[7] but around Astoria it was especially dangerous to healthy Chinese workers. Former Chinese mine workers were healthy and did not endanger other Northwesterners.

---

[6] Washington History Link, encyclopedia, "Smallpox Epidemic of 1862 among Northwest Coast and Puget Sound Indians."
[7] *Astoria Daily Bulletin*, August 16, 1881.

Nineteen years before 1900, local and regional doctors were already acting against smallpox and not waiting for a federal isolation building to be constructed. Their strategy was to dry up the pool of people whom smallpox could infect in the future. On September 15, 1881, smallpox vaccinations were required of school children.[8] Experimental vaccines might do the job and efforts were made to immunize more and more Oregonians. It was hoped that eventually, smallpox would be deprived of potential hosts in one geographical area.

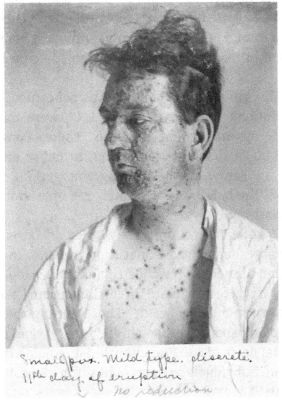

Smallpox. Mild type. discrete.
11th day of eruption
no reduction

Courtesy NAUS, RG 90, Male infected with smallpox.

[8] *Astoria Daily Bulletin*, September 15, 1881, p.3

11

How many parents actually brought their children to a doctor remains an open question. Whether teachers checked for vaccinations inside the classroom is also questionable.

Equally promising was the offer by the Sisters of Providence to open a hospital in Astoria. As early as July 1880, they had come to plan the opening of such an institution. Their intent promised a dramatic improvement in available institutional health care. According to Dr. Leinassar, in 1893, Oregon's medical school was still called a dumping ground for untalented medical professionals who had failed to obtain licenses in other states. Going to the doctor in Oregon was more of a crapshoot than visits in other parts of the nation. For Astorians, only a tiny pest house existed on main street in 1887. The county maintained no pest house at that time.[9]

As far as disease arriving on ships was concerned, Astorians expecting solutions from Washington, D.C., were told to look further north instead to Puget Sound. There, Congress had funded and built a first official building to house dangerously sick passengers. Sadly, for those living and working in Astoria and Knappton, the building was located 275 miles north in Port Townsend, Washington.

There Dr. Samuel M. McCurdy had opened an extremely basic space exuberantly misnamed a maritime hospital. In reality, it was nothing but a crude set of wooden planks nailed together until it was a very large rectangular, three-dimensional box located far outside town in a dense wood.[10] Those putting their trust in words printed on paper advertised in 1887 that it represented the largest hospital north of San Francisco, but it remained a hopeless shack to isolate individuals so they could suffer alone. When an ill

[9] Astoria Public Library, Dr. Jorma Michael Leinassar, *Memoir*, June 16, 1887. Partially based on W. Samuels, *West Shore Magazine*, p.21.
[10] Paula Becker, entry: "Federal Maritime Quarantine Station for Puget Sound," History Lin.org Essay 8203, James G. Mc Curdy in By Juan de Fuca's Strait, on HistoryLink.org, free online encyclopedia of Washington State History, accessed January 18, 2015.

person was quarantined, an old male sailor designated to act as nurse was certainly not a comforting image. A doctor would stop by when he had spare time and patients were told to wait and see if and how they would survive. During those years, the records do not mention any ship with an ill passenger on board transferring from Astoria to Port Townsend.[11]

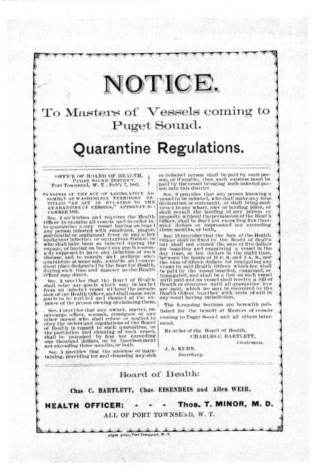

Courtesy Washington State Historical Society, ID: 1997.1.289, Puget Sound Quarantine Regulations, 1882.

[11] Ibid

By then, any ship's passage from Asia to the U.S. also had taken on an additional racial tone. Officially, the 1882 passage of the Chinese Exclusion Act was to dampen any enthusiasm for direct transport of male workers from China. Unofficially, in Astoria, the act was more disregarded than followed and individuals continued to arrive by themselves from China. In particular men skilled in business found sympathetic inspectors in Astoria often willing to differ with their supervisors in Portland and they admitted the transoceanic migrants. Besides, most ship crews arriving from Asia employed large numbers of men certifying as ethnically Chinese.

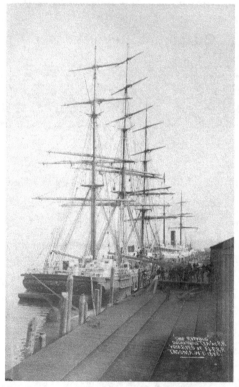

Courtesy Tacoma Public Library, 38263.jpg, Thomas H. Rutter, The "Republic" discharges a load of Asian tea at the North Pacific Railroad wharf and station in Tacoma, 1888.

In May 1888, the Northern Pacific Railroad reached Puget Sound and Tacoma. From now on, transpacific ship-to-rail traffic would take place in the Northwest. In the same month, the owners of the same railroad announced that Astoria and the Columbia River would play no central role in their national infrastructure plans. Instead of choosing the mouth of the nation's second-largest river as the terminus for another northern crossing of the continental nation, they remained content with only their presence in Puget Sound and Tacoma. Astoria would not be a railroad boomtown anytime soon.

Astorian dreams of iron horses bringing business and citizens to the mouth of the Columbia, from where they would transfer to ships ready to cross to Asia, would have to remain pipe dreams and commercial fantasy.

What the arrival of the railroad meant was reported in the news from Tacoma. As Tacoma became the terminus of a transcontinental line linked to a cross Pacific Ocean ship connection, the town rapidly transformed into a city.

Not surprisingly, Congressional representatives soon took action. Congress appropriated federal money to upgrade the quarantine shack near Port Townsend to make it a basic, professional quarantine station. Indeed, an 1888 funding bill asked for $55,000. The total broke down like this: $10,000 was to construct a hospital and quarters for resident officers, a second $10,000 would build a wharf and warehouses where disinfection machines were to be installed at the cost of about $20,000; finally, $500 would purchase a small boat. Annual operating costs were projected to require $10,000.

The upgraded station opened on July 13, 1889. From 1889 to 1891, 535 vessels stopped there and were investigated for dangerous diseases.[12] Elsewhere in the nation, seven other stations

[12] U.S. Surgeon General Report, 1890/1891, p. 14.

15

conducted federally supervised quarantine business.[13] Near the large port of San Francisco, Angel Island opened in 1890.[14]

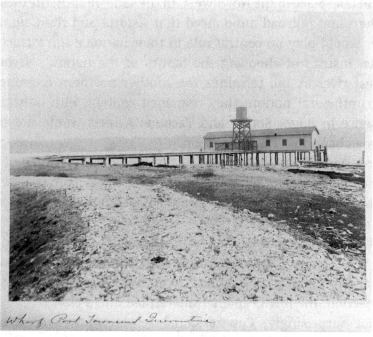

Courtesy NAUS, RG 90, The improved quarantine station at Port Townsend.

Still, politicians in Washington, D.C. were not enthusiastic about opening a quarantine station near Astoria or, at least, about spending money to station their well-educated doctors inside modern equipped medical offices. In essence, political leaders did not believe that health work deserved priority at that location. Even though a noticeable gap in service existed between San Francisco and Port Townsend, leaders lacked the foresight to close that gap and create a seamless West Coast protection service. And thus, this book would almost have closed right here.

[13] They were Cape Charles, Delaware Beachwater, Gulf, Key West, San Diego, San Francisco and South Atlantic.

[14] U.S. Surgeon General Report 1890/1891. Whereas near Seattle 196 ships had been stopped in Angel Island only 46 ships had to be inspected. Four of them had to be disinfected.

What remained in the years thereafter were local people continuing to help themselves to dream, which meant staying focused on business. 1887 was recognized as a banner year for the cannery industry. Finns fished like mad while Chinese stuffed cans according to a merciless rhythm of labor that the industry would insist upon for another century. Ten canneries operated on the Washington side of the river and thirteen on the Oregon side.[15] Nature was mentioned only if it could be described as something that would earn money.

Those conscious of a bigger picture, hoped they themselves would not one day be isolated in a country pest house, condemned to pray and wait to see if they would get well despite the lack of effective federal medicine.

Local doctors tied to Oregon's health service accepted the additional task of vaccinating incoming sailors and passengers. For example, on May 8, 1889, a vessel of the Hong Kong Steamship Company was found to carry a passenger with smallpox. Fortunately, the infected person had been discovered in Honolulu and placed into the island kingdom's quarantine system. Once the ship made it to Astoria, the Oregon state quarantine service quarantined it. Two doctors boarded the vessel and vaccinated those who showed no signs of vaccination. Thereafter they released the ship and it continued up the river.

Remarkable individual doctors who wanted to rise above simply following average bureaucratic principles emerge from the records during this time. They sought and found individual allies in Astoria's maritime culture who shared such an enlightened, inspired outlook. For instance, on the Oregon side, the systematic vaccination of school children was followed up with a public education campaign that trained bar pilots and ship captains.

---

[15] Chart of the Columbia River from the Ocean to Portland Oregon, columbiariverimages. com; p.17.

Ironically, it was nature that nudged federal politicians toward taking new steps to open a station near Astoria. It took the fifth cholera pandemic to force Washington, D.C. policymakers to look beyond their usual spending priorities, who again and again had ranked the need for any Astoria station as low.

Only cholera on U.S. soil created enough pressure to bring together budgets, people, doctors, and merchants from both coasts. Cholera on the East Coast gave renewed credence to those voices that had always argued that the absence of a Columbia station offered dangerous diseases 700 unguarded miles for entry. Between Tacoma and San Francisco, this opening space beckoned nature to take advantage of it, cross it, and savor human hosts on U.S. soil as diseases replicated with renewed appetite.

Vibrio Cholera, the bacteria that causes cholera, had begun its new march across the world in 1881. Month after month, it traveled on from India toward Europe. It was its fifth pandemic in human history and it enthusiastically made use of the infrastructure built by global British colonialism and the first globalization era to hurry its journey.

Of course, eventually it was able to implant itself in the United States as well. Fortunately for Astorians, it arrived first on the East Coast, on boats coming from Europe.[16]

The professionals of the U.S. Marine Hospital Service could track the fifth cholera pandemic. International communication had accelerated enough to have a near real-time notion of what the pandemic was doing. The nation's citizens might not care until they themselves were hemorrhaging vital liquids somewhere on a cot too far away from a doctor to receive help fast.

But the health service's doctors, out of professional pride and institutional self-interest, recognized this pandemic as a

---

[16] Howard Markel, Quarantine! East European Jewish Immigrants and the New York Epidemics of 1892, (Baltimore and London: John Hopkins Press, 1997), p.85.

showcase opportunity to demonstrate how much the nation and its business could benefit from a yet-to-be expanded institutional, federalized health service.

This danger to American life also provided an opportunity to cement the doctor's professional role as part of a federal institution and workforce. Doctors passed the test with flying colors, demonstrating their critical value as they kept cholera from advancing. The majority of citizens had no idea what terrible consequence they had been spared and continued to amuse themselves with whatever was on their mind during those months.

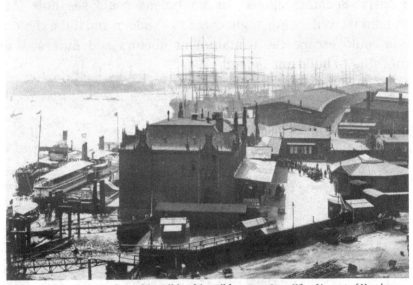

Courtesy Germany, Bundesarchiv, Bildarchiv, Bild 137-107849, *Wharf in port of Hamburg, Germany; emigrants in line to board ship for journey overseas, 1895.*

Of course, it did not hurt that business leaders had also begun to plead for more federal health help. They may not have cared so much about the people, but they certainly cared about their economic expectations from the upcoming World's Columbian

Exposition in Chicago, which might be deflated if millions of
visitors decided not to travel to Chicago from where they might
possibly bring home a life-threatening case of cholera, just
because "they had wanted to encounter the world."

The U.S. public was looking forward to this major national
cultural event. It symbolized how much Americans wanted to
see themselves at the forefront of the first age of globalization.
A cholera outbreak would seriously discourage travel and
participation at the fair. Indeed, a collapse of tourism, it was
feared, could even precipitate a general collapse of the nation's
financial system. Such a financial panic had to be avoided at
all costs, Senators agreed, as politicians could see how U.S.
commercial well-being might come to a sudden end if the cholera
virus could escape the containment doctors and nurses were
promising to build and defend.

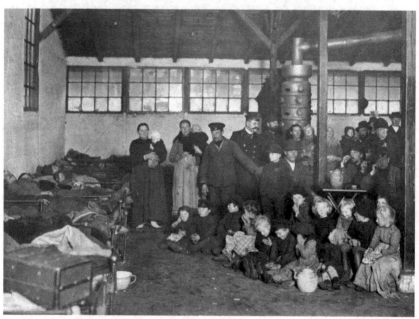

Courtesy Germany Bundesarchiv, Bildarchiv, Bild 137-107845, *Waiting room in port of
Hamburg, Germany, showing emigrants waiting, 1890s.*

In 1891, the U.S. federal government took the right to process its own immigrants from the states. It handed the responsibility of organizing the medical inspection of immigrants from Europe and Asia to the Marine Hospital Service on March 3rd, 1891.

In August, the *Moravia* coming from Hamburg, Germany with 336 passengers on board arrived in New York. That meant 22 less than had left the port of Hamburg. They had died of cholera during the journey and had to be buried at sea. The news of the arrival of cholera in New York quickly made its way up and down the East Coast, causing particularly bad excitement in Boston. As early as October 9, 1891, a first circular letter asked to stop importing rags from France suspected of having been used in European areas where cholera was raging. By August 1892, the stoppage of rag imports became complete, targeting all areas of the world.[17] Most of us have heard of the station opening in front of New York harbor at Ellis Island in 1892. Private companies chipped in as well. Ten dormitories were built at New York's Pier No. 10 on the so-called America Kai. In case of an emergency 1,400 people could be isolated there, housed, and, if possible returned to health.

By then, news from Hamburg reported the deaths of thousands of people, decreasing the population of this large city. The cholera epidemic began to slow the global dispersion of emigrants. Observers in New York reported that ships from Hamburg and Bremen, Germany, arrived surprisingly empty. The number of emigrants crossing the Atlantic in steerage dropped dramatically. Prospective passengers were now being held back at the Polish-German border, long before they ever made it to Hamburg or Bremen to embark.

This cholera pandemic was beginning to endanger the very economic foundations of European transatlantic passenger

[17] U.S. Surgeon General Report 1891/1892, p. 38.

lines. They depended on predictable emigration fares. A U.S. Senate Committee on Immigration even considered suspending immigration altogether for at least 12 months.[18] Such a decision would have forced the collapse of major national shipping lines in Germany, France, the Netherlands, and Great Britain.

So far we have listed only short-term consequences that resulted from the 1892 cholera epidemic. Today, some visitors ask why so few ill people had to stay at the Knappton Cove's Columbia River Quarantine Station. The answer is because of the result of long-term changes initiated by the 1892 cholera pandemic.

The planners reimagined the battlefield of the war against infectious diseases. In 1858, unknown individuals in New York had torched the quarantine building located in the middle of the urban area in order to protest against foolish decision-makers who had placed highly infectious people in the middle of a city. Thereafter, quarantine stations were moved to the edges of urban centers where fewer people lived.

In 1892, the issue came up again: Why let infected people come into the country and stay at the edge of cities? It made more sense to keep them out of the U.S. before they stepped on a boat and until they had recovered. Thus, planners moved the location of the first engagement between global nature and U.S. doctors overseas. The initial perimeter of defense where the opposing forces met was moved back across the ocean, from U.S. ports to European, African, Latin American, and Asian port cities.

In the Pacific, Hawaii, again located outside the U.S. mainland, was elevated in importance. In 1893 a legislative act empowered the U.S. government to quarantine individuals on one island before they reached the U.S. mainland. The very small number of ill people that might still slip through the observations of health

---

[18] Howard Markel, *Quarantine! East European Jewish Immigrants and the New York Epidemics of 1892*, (Baltimore and London: John Hopkins Press, 1997), p.166

officials at Asian ports now could be held in a single, distant locale before making it to U.S. territory. Honolulu became a bulwark of last resort outside the U.S. before ships completed their Pacific crossing and reached San Francisco, Astoria, Oregon, or Tacoma, Washington. Every effort was made to meet the natural enemy at locations outside the U.S. mainland before it could ever replicate inside of it.

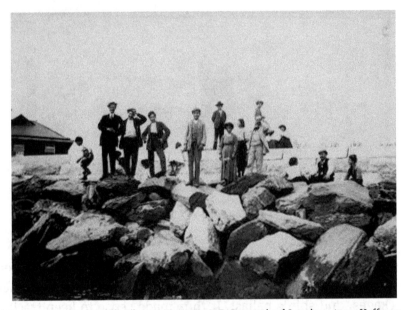

Courtesy New York Public Library, ID # 732083F, Quarantined Immigrants on Hoffman Island, New York's quarantine area.

Doctors reimagined how to gain data about health threats. We all know that dangerous infections can travel inside people. Therefore, a certification system was created that tracked the health of arriving immigrants and passengers. Tracking began with an examination in the country from which they wanted to depart. This work was supervised by a health specialist employed

23

inside a U.S. consulate. A consulate suddenly no longer employed just diplomats, using words to manage politics, but also health specialists, using sight to identify evolving epidemics before they hit our country. In a financially smart move, responsibility for tracking was placed in the hands of private foreign transport companies. Even today, airline companies have to vouch for their passengers.

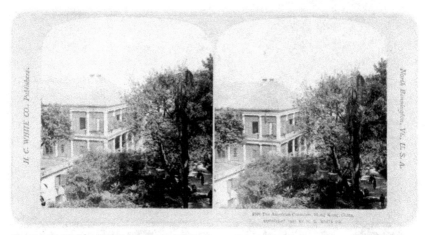

Courtesy LOC, The U.S. Consulate in Hong Kong, China, 1901.

And yet, dangerous infections could also be brought here by other means than human beings, such as luggage, clothes, packages, and ship's ballast. It thus made sense to keep track of those inanimate items in addition to people, so ships were ordered to keep and present a history of its sanitary health. They had to carry a record listing the number of people and their health, plus a cargo list and statements of whether diseases had been present. Not only did immigrants and visitors have to provide a sanitary history, but a ship had to demonstrate its sanitary history as well. Ships and the owners who repeatedly proved inattentive to sanitary issues would quickly catch the attention of health inspectors.

Next, luggage acquired a heightened importance during inspection. Circular No. 141 from August 17, 1892, decreed that all personal items coming from Russia had to be numbered and then disinfected.[19] One week later, Circular No. 147 required that suitcases and personal belongings from Asia and Europe also had to be disinfected. It became an almost universal requirement. Quarantine stations were now no longer about people but also, in their own right, ships and cargo. Just as a human army might attack an enemy with mixed forces, such as infantry, cavalry, and navy, the U.S. Marine Hospital Service deployed specialists, distinguishing between humans, ships, and the items they brought.

Courtesy NAUS, S.S. Batavia, Report of examination, 1892.

[19] U.S. Surgeon General Report 1892/1893, p. 285.

Finally, long-term changes broke the customary political division of domestic political powers. The executive branch gained dictatorial powers when it came to matters of health. U.S. presidents could enforce sanitary rules and stop an individual or cargo from coming onto U.S. soil. Within the country, the U.S. Marine Hospital Service was given unprecedented federal power that could order regional and local government representatives what to do. A new law titled "an act granting additional quarantine powers and imposing additional duties upon the Marine Hospital Service" was signed by President Benjamin Harrison on February 15, 1893.

Overnight, these laws added to the role of the Marine Hospital Service doctors' power to become someone who could wield political power in regions and local cities. In a health emergency, local and regional elected officials had to obey instructions from somebody who had not been elected by the people they wanted to protect.

Through matters of health, the power of the federal government and how far from Washington D.C. it could exercise it became visible. Previously, this has been the case only when national elections were held or in a case of military importance. If a station should ever be built in Astoria, the doctors representing the U.S.M.H.S. could give orders to Oregon politicians and the mayor of Astoria. Cholera indirectly shifted the distribution of domestic political powers.

After relocating the initial fight between U.S. doctors and natural infection to overseas locations, and changing expectations of who could order whom in a health emergency domestically, the 1892 epidemic opened a flow of federal money to cities on both coasts. Finally, real construction of new and expanded quarantine stations replaced mere words in rule books.

Along the West Coast, in San Diego, a new wharf was built, plus a warehouse and a new hospital. Finally, a simple but sturdy gangway connected the station with the shore. In front of San Francisco, a federal quarantine station was built. At Ayalo Cove foreign ships were already being fumigated and travelers isolated, should they have arrived carrying diseases. Now a federal building and presence was constructed at Angel Island. Until its opening, the U.S. Navy placed the U.S.S. *Omaha* there. In 1893, its facilities supplied overheated steam for fumigation.[20] A second steamer was also anchored there and refurbished to function as a disinfection building. *The George M. Sternberg* made available the latest technology and chemicals ready to kill viruses and bacteria inside people, clothes, suitcases, and cargo.

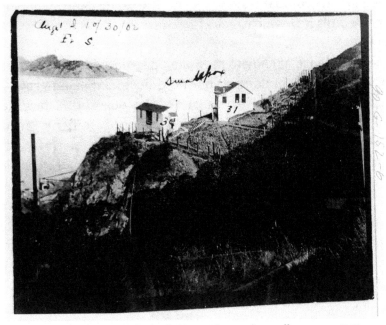

Courtesy NAUS, RG 90, Angel Island, CA, pest houses for smallpox cases, 1902.

[20] California Department of Parks and Recreation, accessed January, 29, 2015

In Astoria, Oregon, a federal health presence had still not appeared by 1893. Once again, Astorians were told to tow and sail their infected people to Port Townsend. In Puget Sound, the quarantine station was radically modernized. A committee staffed by a customs officer, a surgeon, and a physician identified 153 acres as appropriate for purchase costing $3500.[21] On March 3, 1893, federal funds were authorized to move the quarantine station from Challam Point to Diamond Point. By November, the growing federal presence presented 27 new buildings that replaced the three shacks for hopeless sufferers. Now, infected people could be treated more humanely and professionally, helped by the existence of a new wharf, a warehouse, a hospital, a laundry building, and quarters for a surgeon general.[22]

Even private companies chipped in. The Pacific Mail Steamship Company built its own barracks there offering beds for up to 500 people.[23]

The experience of cholera in 1892 had replaced hope, talk, and paper with federal buildings and more doctors. Such a growing presence and the new powers of federal quarantine facilities still begged the question of future quarantine stations run by the states of California, Oregon, and Washington. However, the resulting tensions would not turn into open, vehement conflict for a few more years.

During this time on the West Coast, diseases other than cholera kept doctors and city leaders on edge. Smallpox, cholera's co-conspirator in death, sent 25 people to Angel Island's quarantine station between October 1891 and 1892. Twice it was able to defeat the doctors and killed an infected patient.

---

[21] U.S. Surgeon General Report, p. 85.
[22] U.S. Surgeon General Annual Report 1892/1893, p. 259.
[23] U.S. Surgeon General Report, p. 56.

Most importantly, smallpox was never just a challenge from Asia. While the Grim Reaper sailed in from China, in December 1891, two months later, it tried to breach U.S. defenses from the south, coming from Rio de Janeiro, Brazil. Because these few cases had been caught and citizens were successfully protected, human journeys across the Pacific only increased. Of course, the need to inspect also increased in those years. In 1892, the number of foreign arrivals in Puget Sound surpassed those in San Francisco. There, the public health service inspected 282 ships and passed their cargo while Angel Island handled only 53 vessels. In Puget Sound only 7 vessels had to be detained and disinfected.[24] Angel Island quarantined 53 vessels and inspected 15 additional ones.[25]

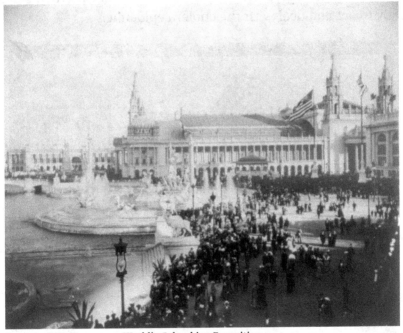

Courtesy LOC, Panorama, World's Columbian Exposition.

[24] U.S. Surgeon General, report 1891/1892.
[25] U.S. Surgeon General report 1892, p. 56.

Of course, the World's Columbian Exposition also opened as planned. It would enter history books as a place where people, filled with wonder, excitedly watched presentations, not a place where they picked up a case of a life-threatening, most horrible disease like cholera. "The show went on," while earnest doctors and nurses did their utmost to allow this commercial dream to be dreamed, and they largely succeeded. The 1892 epidemic never materialized inside the U.S. The infection left the U.S. and continued on other continents.

Reports to Washington D.C. attested to how valiantly the men and the women of the U.S. Marine Hospital Service had performed. The U.S.M.H.S. had demonstrated the value of its techniques, scientific knowledge, and specialists. They had shown themselves ready to act and deal with the cholera epidemic.

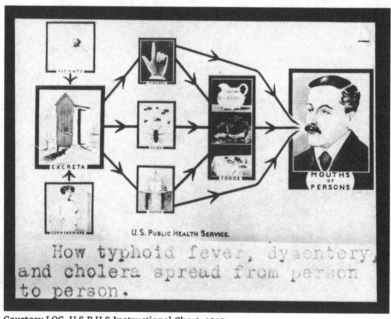

Courtesy LOC, U.S.P.H.S Instructional Chart, 1910.

They had confronted and stopped the real and immense danger and experience of cholera cases on U.S. soil. U.S. lawmakers were presented with a heroic story as they contemplated voting for more federal funds for the service. After the cholera of 1892, the U.S.M.H.S. had a proven track record as a highly valuable national institution that deserved praise and, most importantly, more funds to grow in service to the nation.

Against this backdrop, the absence of a quarantine station at the mouth of the nation's second-largest river finally became more and more difficult to justify. At the very least, logic suggested that the Columbia River should also have such a federal defense health outpost.

In 1894, local Astorians, international shipping companies, and their Oregon political representatives finally mustered enough clout to enter a bill in the U.S. Congress. With the scare of 1892, fresh in their minds, a first request for funds for an Astoria quarantine station was attached to a sundry appropriation bill in the U.S. Congress in Washington, D.C., in March 1894.

That same year, the third Grim Reaper *yersinia pestis* or, in English, the plague, began the third year of its fifth journey around the world in the last thousand years. Starting in 1892, it was using the movements of soldiers and trade up and down the Yangtze River with great success, always finding new human hosts.

The pickings were rich. In March 1894, the plague ravaged 60,000 people. In April and May, the total continued to grow, another 40,000 people had to be buried. Yet, despite this obvious observable cavalcade of death, regular ship traffic from Canton to Hong Kong never stopped. What's more, in Hong Kong, captains continued to bet that they could earn money without being impacted by the approaching plague, deceiving themselves they could carry only healthy people and cargo across the Pacific to San Francisco or Tacoma, interrupted by only a short stop over in Honolulu.

Friedrich E. Schuler

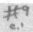

53D CONGRESS, }   SENATE.   { EX. DOC.
2d Session. }   { No. 130.

IN THE SENATE OF THE UNITED STATES.

LETTER

FROM

THE SECRETARY OF THE TREASURY,

IN RESPONSE TO

The Senate resolution of June 26, 1894, transmitting copies of correspondence and reports concerning the importance of and urgency for the establishment of a quarantine station at or near the mouth of the Columbia River, and stating what action is necessary thereto.

JULY 9, 1894.—Referred to the Committee on Appropriations and ordered to be printed.

TREASURY DEPARTMENT,
OFFICE OF THE SECRETARY,
Washington, D. C., July 7, 1894.

SIR: I have the honor to acknowledge receipt of Senate resolution of the 26th instant directing that there be transmitted to the Senate copies of all correspondence and reports and all information in the possession of this Department concerning the importance of and urgency for the establishment of a quarantine hospital at or near the mouth of the Columbia River, and to inform the Senate whether any Congressional action is necessary concerning the same.

In reply I have to transmit herewith a letter from the Supervising Surgeon-General of the Marine-Hospital Service, together with a copy of the report by Passed Assistant Surgeon James B. Stoner, of the Marine-Hospital Service, upon the quarantine administration and facilities at the port of Astoria at the mouth of the Columbia River. Also a copy of a letter addressed from this Department to the collector of customs at Astoria, Oreg., giving instructions concerning the course to be pursued in the event of the arrival of an infected vessel at that port.

From the papers inclosed it will be observed that while a careful inspection is maintained at the port of Astoria, there is no provision there for the removal of the sick from an infected vessel nor for the vessel's disinfection. An infected vessel, under the circumstances, would necessarily be sent to the national quarantine station near Port Townsend, some 275 miles distant.

If, in view of the increasing commerce of the port of Astoria, as well as its present commercial importance and the great distance from the nearest disinfection station, it is deemed necessary to establish this station, a Congressional appropriation, not to exceed $40,000, should be

Courtesy Clatsop County Historical Society, Astoria, Oregon, Letter, U.S. Secretary of State answering Senate Resolution June 16, 1894.

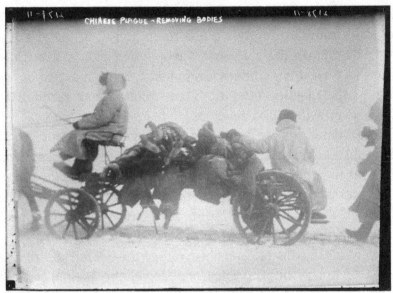

Courtesy LOC, Plague in China; removal of the dead.

The professionals of the U.S.M.H.S. were aware of the terrifying advance of *yersinia pestis*. Thanks to the reforms of 1892, the service delivered intelligence updates, only its focus was not terrorism or religious zealotry but the mingling of virus, bacteria, and humans. In Washington, D.C., where the reports were gathered and analyzed, they became a constant ominous drumbeat in the background as debates for and against a station in Astoria continued without any resolution in sight. Doctors of the U.S.M.H.S. did not have the slightest doubt that plague would be delighted to replicate inside Oregonians and Washingtonians if their travel and commercial desires, however, opened the Northwest to it.

Key voices in Astoria, however, did not share that outlook. Instead of echoing the resounding plea to "spare humans from the plague" being chanted by health professionals, they offered the more upbeat chorus that business income should be protected from slowing down due to an arrival of plague. They were whistling in the dark that it would be a shame if business in the Northwest would deteriorate just because a single patient carrying the plague, unquarantined, might break through the otherwise effective 1892 defenses.

Most did not prepare at all for a battle against the Grim Reaper that could be arriving at any time. Local advocates for a quarantine station at the Columbia, lawmakers in Washington, D.C., and the U.S. executive thus waited another five years until federal money was found to build such a station or to buy an existing suitable building.

Except for the doctors and observers of the U.S.M.H.S., all sides were afflicted by hubris. They banked on the alleged patience of the gods that the plague that was traveling through China, Indochina, and India would not float up on the West Coast anytime soon. But, of course, it did, in 1900. San Franciscans can tell quite a story about this awful miscalculation regarding nature.

In the end, the station for Astoria did at last come. It came here because it was talked into existence as a needed but still lacking symbol of Astorian's commercial greatness. All the other large U.S. commercial port cities counted such a station within their bays and only Astoria did not have one yet, it was argued.

The five years between 1894 and 1899 offer another example of how too many experts failed to pay the eternal respect due to nature. That Astorians were not ravaged by plague was luck, but never a confirmation that they could control nature should the plague come early.

The period between 1894 and 1899 was marked by a political, and commercial propaganda effort, arguing that any great port engaging in transpacific or transatlantic trade had to have one station where dangerously diseased passengers could be kept away from others for a month.

This argument did not ask for a three-dimensional building in order to help Astorians or Washingtonians to stay healthy, but because it would upgrade and validate the activity going on at the port, much as with the quarantine stations in San Diego, Port Townsend, New Orleans, Havana, Charleston, or Baltimore. Having a station said that this was a serious port and part of the global maritime interchange.

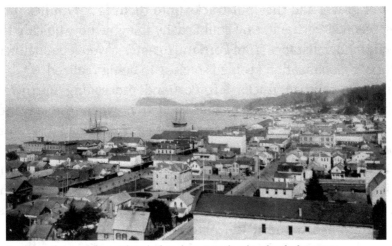

Courtesy Clatsop County Historical Society, Astoria, city view before 1900.

Astorians and their representatives in Congress wanted to see themselves as up-and-coming West Coast and transoceanic traders. Therefore, the argument went, they deserved respect from Washington, D.C., lawmakers and could no longer endure an absence of a station. It was no longer acceptable to send their diseased to Port Townsend.

In the meantime, representatives of the U.S.M.H.S. published updates tracking the approach of the plague, but it played no role in the surviving letters and cables of participating politicians.

For more than a decade, Astorian business and trade circles had insisted that their town was up and coming commercially. Anytime now, railroad construction would reach Astoria and connect this port city with the same iron tracks advancing elsewhere across the nation. Once that happened, it could also connect with a transpacific shipping line to Asia.

The Northern Pacific Railroad had reached Walla Walla, Washington as planned, in 1883. Soon thereafter, a railroad bridge was constructed across the Columbia. Workers kept advancing beds of gravel and they put tracks onto them for 217 miles until they reached Portland. One could easily imagine how quickly the much smaller distance from Portland to Astoria would be spanned. Astoria's globalization seemed so close to being realized.

Indeed, railroad tracks left Portland proceeding northwest along the Columbia River. But suddenly, when the advance reached a location named Goble, Oregon, railroad investors proclaimed that they had run out of money.

True to our American insistence on dreaming, men made up their minds that they would bring the meeting point nearer the sea to Astoria in their view, the logical place. As early as August 1877, they had founded the Astoria & South Coast Railway. A first spike had been driven into the ground on May 11, 1889, at Skipanon. Rail construction had begun in Hillsboro as well.

It did not help. From then on, not a single additional iron rail moved forward to give Astorian dreamers the scenario they sought. After the shock, they had to admit that Portland, the meeting point of the transcontinental Northern Pacific and Union Pacific Railroads would remain the premier location and city in the Northwest.

Thereafter, railroad investors kept voting against spending more investor money to clear brush along the river to lay the missing tracks to the Pacific. In addition, they blew a verbal smoke screen. They argued that, on second look, the Almighty already had created an excellent alternative. God and nature had scratched a very wide river next to where a railroad was imagined to advance. Astorians should see and appreciate the Columbia for what it was: a finished watery slide on which barges could steam downstream and export from Portland whatever Oregonians chose. Astorians simply had to realize that they should invest in iron ships to connect with the Pacific, not in locomotives and flatbed railroad cars.

Historian Leslie M. Scott reminds us of the words that rail investor Villard uttered when he discussed the question of whether Astoria truly needed to be connected with a railroad the way Tacoma or San Francisco were:

> "the [Astoria] railroad was not essential; the Columbia River channel to Portland was cheaper for transport and shortened railroad construction mileage."[26]

International investors also did not care that Astorian dreams had been abandoned "railroad wise," just 60 miles out of town.

Businessmen living in Astoria, even those with connections to San Francisco or Seattle, nonetheless still possessed a million molecules of hope and entrepreneurial itch. Unfortunately for them they could not present millions of dollars to fund tracks. No Warren Buffett-like personality lived in Astoria who might easily and happily have wanted to fill the financial void, covering the blemish on the city's commercial imagination.

In the end, all that Astorians could do was to keep on nourishing an abortive longing that invited men to dream too big, in this case, the dream of an elusive investor who wanted to see and pay for a railroad that could be connected to transpacific shipping lines.

[26] Leslie M. Scott, 226.

A few well-to-do Astorian citizens attempted a form of local grandeur. Captain Flavel made land available at today's value of $8.2 million.[27] The Flavel Land and Development Company was incorporated in Salem and charged with building a railroad from Salem, via Sheridan and Tillamook, until it would reach the town of Flavel, only miles away from Astoria.

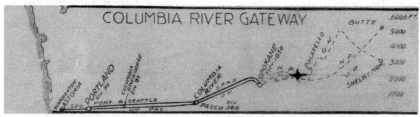

Courtesy Warrenton Tourist Info, Wishful thinking: Astoria rail to transpacific ship connection.

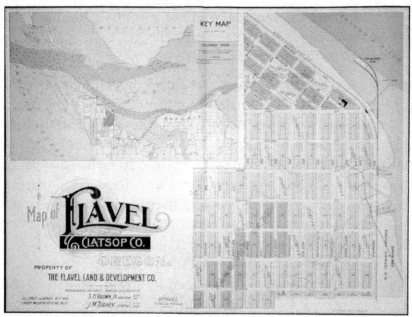

Courtesy Clatsop County Historical Society, Wishful thinking: Flavel a town that was never built.

[27] 2014 value based on conversion table dave.com; a 1896 court record mentions the assumed foreclosure value of $315,000. 1 Dollar in 1892 equals 26.32 in 2014.

Plans from 1893 show on paper a pier that offered a rail-to-ship connection.[28] It might not connect across the Pacific but at least to San Francisco. Some local dreamers even saw the town of Flavel rivaling the sister city of Astoria. Who knew, perhaps, it might become the town that shipping lines would choose as the final destination, steaming in from Honolulu, Hawaii.

Then, reality showed its face. For the next five years, the company's shareholders failed to make payments so that in 1896 the property was foreclosed.[29] Still a nice hotel was being built for well-to-do travelers who could afford to stay at a fine place overlooking the coast and the ocean. By the end of the 19th century, the town of Flavel rivaled nothing and nobody, and the railroad from Tillamook never made it north. As for the railroad from Portland, it still ended in Goble, where all passengers had to switch to a sternwheeler or climb into a horse drawn-buggy to endure the bumpy ride on a dirt road, very poorly cushioned by the four leather strips mounted on the sides of the wagon. As far as health was concerned, the U.S. Collector of Customs and head of Astoria's ironwork John Fox lamented:

> "but there is still no provision to remove such people from an infected vessel, nor the ability to disinfect the vessel. Right now a ship with infected crew or passengers would have to be sent to the only existing quarantine station. However, it was located 275 miles north of the mouth of Columbia at Port Townsend."[30]

But up in Tacoma, railroad dreams had become reality, and the opening of a transcontinental railroad terminus was transforming the previously unimportant place into a boomtown.

[28] February 24, 1893, J.M. Turney, pa 35-37, February 24 1893. James Morris Turney described himself in a yearbook of Yale as "Boomer of Flavel."
[29] San Francisco Call, Vol. 80, Number 69, August 8, 1896.
[30] NAUS, (National Archive of the United States), Central File, 1897-1923, RG 90, Letter, J.G. Carlisle Secretary to President of the U.S. Senate, July 7, 1894.

By 1890, Tacoma's population had grown to 30,000 residents. Still further north, in Everett, the arrival of the Great Northern Railroad in 1893 brought the boom that Astorian commercial circles so craved.

Unfortunately, what happened further north did not rub off on Astoria. The stubborn absence of a railroad terminus kept the port uninteresting for ocean crossings and more isolated than it had to be.

What was uninteresting for investors remained tempting for nature to probe. For example, between 1891 and 1892 at Angel Island, doctors pulled 25 individuals sick with smallpox from incoming foreign ships. Two of the patients died in quarantine. Luckily, no cases were reported in Astoria. Nevertheless, ships continued to transport dangerous diseases to the West Coast.[31]

Instead of plugging the gap in the human-made defense perimeter by establishing a station, people only sent paper with ink to an inbox in Congress, asking for help. And yet, submitting written comments symbolized real progress. The professionals of the federal service were nudging forward regular citizens ignorant of biology and therefore more confused over how to bring about change.

In 1894, it was officials of the national health service who led the petitioning in Congress. That meant they were able to win an unknown sponsor who agreed to attach their petition to his bill and make the request of $40,000 for a station at the mouth of the Columbia.[32] It was thus a doctor who had banged on Congress' door, not a railroad baron, a shipping magnate, or the mayor of Astoria.

[31] U.S. Surgeon General report 1891/1892, p. 56.
[32] NAUS, RG 90, Central File, 1897-1923, Report, Author Walter Wyman, to Asst Surgeon J B Stoner, May 8, 1894.

In May 1894, Assistant Secretary of Health Stoner spelled out for the first time what a quarantine station should look like: a pier, one warehouse, one steam disinfection chamber, a surplus fumigating furnace, tanks for holding ship's ballast, a small hospital, quarters for officers and men, a boat house, and a boarding vessel. His description asked for an ideal arrangement, not reality. Today, when you look outside the windows of the lazaretto's isolation area at Knappton Cove, you see that most of what he described was never built. More about this in the second volume of this series.

He had asked for $1,070,860 in 2014 dollars. No other private investor in 1895 promised to send a larger influx of money into the bay. Only the most financially cognizant realized that the establishment of a federal health presence would also create a new economic center of gravity. Its magnetism would radiate differently from the dizzy money of railroad promoters that was there one day and, inexplicably, gone the next, or the small packet of cash and savings local business owners brought to the town's table.[33] The arrival of the federal health service meant not only real, tangible, physical protection from the plague, and unwelcomed rivalry for Oregon's state-licensed doctors, but also a cool, fresh, delicious flush of greenbacks into local businesses, still surrounded as they sometimes were by mossy stumps from first growth trees that had been cut not too long ago. After all, local stores would have to equip a station with stationery and ink, cut the lumber that held up the roof under which suitcases would await fumigation, and deliver the coal to heat the examination room but only if, finally, Congress could just see the point, pay for it, and build it.

---

[33] NAUS, RG 90, Central File, 1897-1923, Report, Author Walter Wyman, to Asst Surgeon J B Stoner, May 8 1894. This is the 2014 inflation adjusted amount equaling $40,000.

Just as due to the presence of a military base, the purchasing power of newly present officers and rank and file soldiers meant additional city income and community jobs. A federal health presence would mean an uptick in local payroll and noticeably more demand for some select products.[34] In other words, federal health service there also would bring financial health.

There must have existed broader support for Astoria beyond the one individual sponsor who had introduced the bill because the bill made it to the Senate. On June 26, a Senate resolution asked all interested parties to provide "all correspondence and report information about importance and urgency of establishment of a quarantine hospital at or near the mouth of the Columbia." Any new material would provide additional support for Assistant Secretary Stoner's effort.[35]

This health service representative added urgency to the slow political process. Just as in San Francisco, he argued, the establishment of services in Astoria could be accelerated by towing an old navy vessel to Astoria and in 1895 to open it as a temporary place to sequester people or disinfect luggage.

Interestingly, the main reason put forward by supporters remained trade, not health. Treasury Secretary J.C. Carlisle wrote to the president of the Senate on July 7,1894, that an increase in commerce in Astoria would justify a station.[36]

The bill survived in the Senate and was sent on to conference for reconciliation with a House bill. There, the hopeful story crashed, again. The bill died in committee. The historical sources do not tell us why.[37]

---

[34] NAUS, RG 90, Central File, 1897-1923, Report, part of report from U.S. Senate, March 7, 1896. Senate asked for $ 269,000 dollars more.
[35] NAUS, RG 90, Central File, 1897-1923, Letter, June 26, 1894.
[36] NAUS, RG 90, Central File, 1897-1923, Letter, Treasury Secretary J.C. Carlisle to the President of the U.S. Senate, Washington, D.C. July 7, 1894.
[37] NAUS, RG 90, Central File, 1897-1923, report, part of report from U.S. Senate, March 7 1896.

From the vantage point of Washington, D.C., and as far as national legislative life was concerned, the bill's death was nothing unusual, not even anything negative. Seldom did a bill survive political horse-trading the first time after its introduction.[38] Political insiders might even have insisted that it should be immediately proposed again as soon as the next legislative cycle.

The way humans dealt with each other in politics thus handed nature a renewed extension during which it could exploit the open mouth of the river. The shifting sands of the Columbia would be no match for the shifty tactics of microbes still eager to find just one more new host to stay alive. Astoria remained a continued scary weakness in the defenses humans attempted to put up along the West Coast as they wrestled with the globalization of plague.

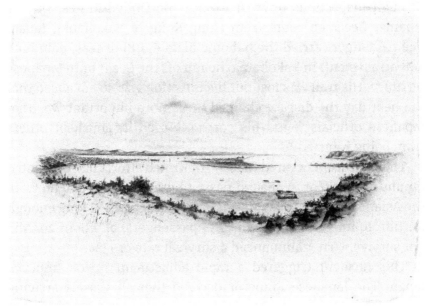

Courtesy LOC, San Diego Bay, 1895.

[38] NAUS, RG 90, Central File, 1897-1923, Letter, Treasury Secretary J.C. Carlisle to the President of the U.S. Senate, Wash, July 7, 1894.

Only a superficial look at 1895 suggested that U.S. defenses were adequate and holding. Far to the south of Astoria, in San Diego, not a single infected passenger had to be treated that year. That meant the health service professionals had managed to pull infected people off boats before their departure from Havana, Cuba, or Callao, Peru, or Manzanilla, Mexico. To the north of Astoria, in Port Townsend not a single infected person had to be quarantined in 1895 either. Again, U.S. medical professionals in Asian ports had paid excellent attention whenever passengers had lined up on wharfs.

Still, insiders knew that plague was creating an explosive spread on the other side of the Pacific and might be able to breach the first U.S. perimeter so valiantly maintained in Asian ports. In 1895, one single person was able to carry the deadly strain through inspections onward toward the United States. On the steamer *Gaelic* en route from Hong Kong to Yokohama, Japan, one passenger carried the bubonic plague, full of fear, pain, and embarrassment. In Yokohama, he ran off the *Gaelic* onto Japanese territory. His trail was lost but his infection was so advanced that the next day the disease claimed him. More important was that Japanese officials found his corpse, buried it, and kept others from being infected.[39]

Then, an event occured that concentrated efforts had prevented up until that point. A second passenger carried the plague from the Asian mainland to Japan. His ship journey lasted long enough for him to infect the crew and 234 passengers, of whom 204 did not survive.[40] That announced a survival rate of 13%!

This incident triggered a rapid adjustment inside Imperial Japan. The Japanese Emperor decreed that all vessels arriving

[39] U.S. Surgeon General report, 1895, p. 546. Not to be forgotten, also one case of smallpox made it from Asia into Japan.
[40] U.S. Surgeon General, Annual report 1895/1896, p.420.

from Hong Kong had to undergo the strictest, most rigid inspections. Moreover, any person suspected in the slightest of being a carrier was locked away into quarantine for seven days. In this way, the Imperial Japanese Health System had indirectly joined the U.S.M.H.S' effort. The U.S. Surgeon General also upped vigilance, stationing another U.S. health officer in Yokohama, Japan. Thus the Japanese port from where most ships crossed the Pacific to Hawaii before reaching Los Angeles, San Francisco, Astoria, Seattle, or Vancouver, Canada had gained an additional set of eyes.[41]

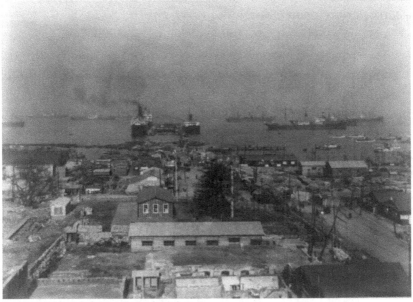

Courtesy LOC, Yokohama, Japan, bay view.

Even so, the news did not improve. In 1896, individuals lucky enough to get their hands on a printed U.S. Surgeon General report read that the plague had reached Hong Kong and on its march there from Canton, it had devoured the next 40,000 individuals.

[41] Ibid. p. 342.

Until the plague arrived in the U.S., however, there was more energy and time to engage in culture wars. In addition to racism, these years added the political dimension of bureaucratic turf wars to health work. Power struggles raged between regional and state professionals and national health service employees over who was in charge.

The law was clear. It asserted federal supremacy over state-based health forces. Still, people at the local level were slow to accept the loss of state authority at their ports. Political battles between state and federal representatives always remained part of the preparations for when the plague would break through the second perimeter in Hawaii and reach the West Coast.

In San Francisco City Hall politicians and the public waged intense debates. Private steamship companies sided with the federal government and the San Francisco Chamber of Commerce voted in favor of cutting the powers of health officials certified by the state of California.[42] In Port Townsend, Tacoma, and Seattle, local representatives kept up the rivalry with federal officers battling over turf, budgets, paid positions, and what buildings to construct.[43]

Of course, in Astoria too, state representatives resented the federal presence. This clash broke into the open only in 1905 when a man called Oswald West, who would become Oregon's governor in the next decade, successfully conspired with the U.S. Marine Hospital Service representative and closed down Oregon's state-run quarantine stations.[44]

§§§

[42] U.S. Surgeon General Report, 1894/1895, p. 308.
[43] Ibid.
[44] NAUS, RG 90, Central File, 1897-1923, Report, part of report from U.S. Senate, March 7, 1896. Thus stations by the State of Oregon remained open in Coos Bay, Gardiner, Yaquina City, Astoria, and Portland. U.S. Surgeon General Report, 914-921.

This was the context within which the leaders of the U.S.M.H.S., backed by Oregon politicians, revived their joint effort in Congress to obtain federal funding for a Columbia River quarantine station. In 1896, a second attempt was started.

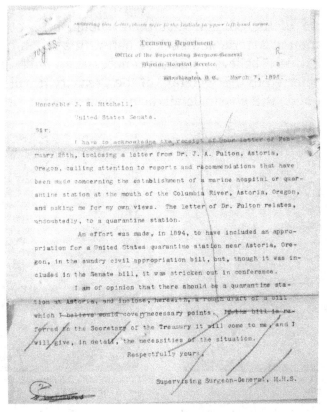

Courtesy NAUS, draft letter, U.S. Surgeon General Walter Wyman to Senator J.H. Mitchell, 1896.

This time an Oregon senator figured prominently alongside the officials of the U.S.M.H.S. Senator J.H. Mitchell was a highly creative individual and a maverick within his Oregon Republican Party. He dominated politics in Portland and Multnomah County. Mitchell cooperated with U.S. Surgeon General Walter Wyman.

On February 25, 1896, Mitchell wrote to Wyman to inquire how he felt about opening a station. It took only 10 days for Wyman to write his reply and to carry it across Pennsylvania Avenue to the Senator's office. On March 7, 1896, Wyman affirmed:

> I am of the opinion that there should be a quarantine station at Astoria and enclose herewith a rough draft of a bill which I believe would cover necessary points. If the bill is referred to the Secretary of the Treasury it will come to me and I will give in detail the necessities of the situation.[45]

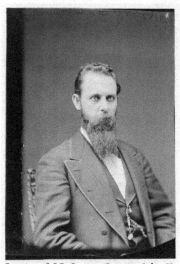

Courtesy LOC, Oregon Senator John H. Mitchell.

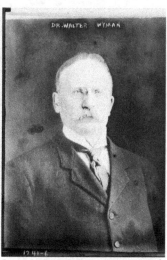

Courtesy LOC, U.S. Surgeon General Dr. Walter Wyman.

Health administrators and national politicians together thus began a second effort to fill the gap at the mouth of the distant river.

On March 23, the Senate Committee on Commerce proposed bill S. 2487 to "require the Secretary of the Treasury to supply all relevant arguments and evidence to decide on passage." An aide

[45] NAUS, RG 90, Central File, 1897–1923, Supervising Surgeon General MHS to Senator J.H.Mitchell, U.S. Senate. March7, 1896.

must have walked the bill down to the Department of the Treasury the same day, because by the next day Treasury administrators were asked to add their documentation.[46] Next, the administrators discussed how best to use the legislative process to obtain funding. In a separate hand-written note, it was suggested that "it would be more advisable to have the matter offered as an amendment to the sundry civil appropriation bill." At this point, the proposal already included a draft form to amend. The submitted bill asked "for the establishment of a quarantine station at or near Astoria, Oregon, for the fiscal year ending June 30, 1897."

The second proposal also suggested, as a temporary measure, to tow a decommissioned U.S. Navy ship into the bay to serve as a floating station where individuals and luggage could be quarantined in an emergency.

The bill did not contemplate buying or refurbishing an existing building, nor did it specify if the station should be located in Oregon or Washington waters. What mattered was that it should be stationed "at or near Astoria." The Senate was presented with a request for $50,000 dollars, the equivalent of $1,070,860 Million today.[47]

Senate Bill S. 966 was read and debated twice in the Committee on Commerce. Then, suddenly, at the end of March, all discussion ceased. Momentum by all sides halted again and nine months of inaction followed. The sources do not explain why.

The standstill in Washington, D.C. contrasted with the explosion of the plague in various populations across the Pacific Ocean. Health specialists reported a quasi-catastrophic situation developing in Hong Kong. On March 2, 1896, a U.S. health observer

[46] NAUS, RG 90, Central File, 1897-1923, Committee on Commerce, U.S. Senate, March 23rd 1896. Carlisle, Secretary of Treasury March 23rd, 1896.
[47] NAUS, Central File, 1897-1923, Report, part of report from U.S. Senate, March 7, 1896 and S 2487, March 23, 1896.

reported that individuals sick with plague were no longer isolated. Free to roam within the healthy population of Hong Kong, plague could now disregard civilization and feast freely. A second report suggested that the situation in Hong Kong was almost as bad as that in Canton. Rumor had it that in Amoy,[48] as well, plague was openly spreading. Officials continued to repress such news in order to protect business.[49]

Inaction around Astoria contrasted with the busy but relatively calm preparations in Angel Island and Port Townsend. There, officials were preparing for the plague to breach the second perimeter ports in Japan and Hawaii and to show up soon inside U.S. port cities.

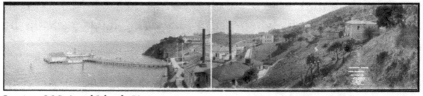

Courtesy LOC, Angel Island, CA.

Two new detention halls were being built near Tacoma providing space for up to 250 passengers at one time.[50] That was only half the size of the halls being built near San Francisco. At Angel Island, two barracks were constructed that could shelter up to 576 passengers. They were linked to a very large disinfection chamber, measuring 50 by 6 feet. There, clothes would be steamed.

In Port Townsend, barracks were constructed for passengers from the entire world. Their presence was not yet attached to a single ethnicity and not called "Philippine, Japanese, or Chinese barracks." In San Francisco, however, people named the wooden retainers the "Chinese barracks."

[48] Today the city is called Xiamin.
[49] U.S. Surgeon General, Annual Report, March 2, 1896 report. Hong Kong. p. 419.
[50] U.S. Surgeon General, Annual Report, p. 308.

The ignorant among us frequently reintroduce the poisonous, mistaken idea that health is an expression of ethnicity or "race." It is not now, never has been, and never will be. Health, people, and nature are part of one and the same global biological process. It was thus wrong to peg this fifth pandemic exclusively onto individuals from Southern China. They were just the first victims of this fifth global battle in the unresolved war called "plague versus homo sapiens" ebbing and flaring up for more than a thousand years.

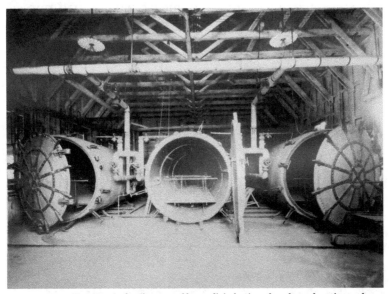

Courtesy NAUS, RG 90, Example of group of large disinfection chambers, location unknown.

Inactivity in Washington, D.C. finally ended on December 10, 1896, when the Senate Committee on Commerce wrote to the Secretary of the Treasury and demanded "attention to the fact that no reply has been received from your department to the letter from the clerk of the committee dated March 23rd, 1896, requesting the views of the Department in relations to the Senate

Bill 2487."[51] No appropriation had been made, and in 1897 no station would rise out of the ground near Astoria. What 1897 would bring remained unclear.[52]

Further north, colonial officials in British Columbia and Vancouver Island had by now joined U.S. colleagues near Tacoma. As passengers walked toward the showers, health inspectors purposely focused on whether travelers showed glandular swelling or open sores. The shower was as much an effort to destroy bacteria through the application of soap as it was a staged walk past U.S. doctors, now on the U.S. mainland, to see quickly, if their colleagues in Hong Kong and Yokohama had missed an infected human being walking by.[53]

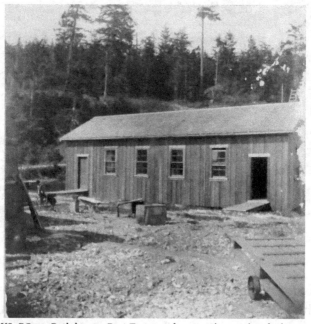

Courtesy NAUS, RG 90, Bath house, Port Townsend quarantine station during construction.

[51] NAUS, RG 90, Central File, 1897-1923, Letter, Committee on Commerce to Secretary of the Treasury, Clerk Woodbury Pulsifer, December 10, 1896.
[52] NAUS, RG 90, Central File, 1897-1923, Supervising Surgeon General to J.H. Mitchell, U.S. Senate, March 7 , 1896.
[53] U.S. Surgeon General, Annual report 1895/1896.

At that point individuals asked to bathe in Port Townsend were receiving no clothes during the disinfection process and had to wait covered up only in anything they could find.

Therefore, the administrators asked Washington, D.C., for 100 suits. Sometimes the bathing of steerage passengers still meant little more than hosing them down with a hose connected to a force pump.[54] Finally, administrators requested installation of a 10-mile long telephone line to speed up communication.

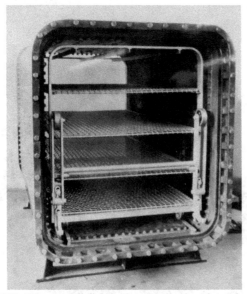

Courtesy NAUS, RG 90, Small disinfection steamer, location unknown.

In Angel Island, trunks were now placed next to smoldering sulfur pots for 24 hours. Their contents could be opened by authorities and select articles were steamed for 30 minutes at 212 degrees. By then, the Canadian Pacific Company was refusing to transport certain types of cargo coming from China. French steamship companies stopped transporting people from Chinese ports altogether. The advancing plague was beginning to change

[54] Ibid, 554.

53

how people and things crossing the Pacific were seen and treated, just as cholera crossing the Atlantic had brought deep changes in 1892.

Nobody knew what would happen if plague made it to Tacoma. Insiders admitted that in case of an infection the best option was probably to run away to avoid being infected.[55] That would mean that the barracks and the infected individuals would no longer be guarded and instead, be left to their own devices able to spread onto U.S. soil.

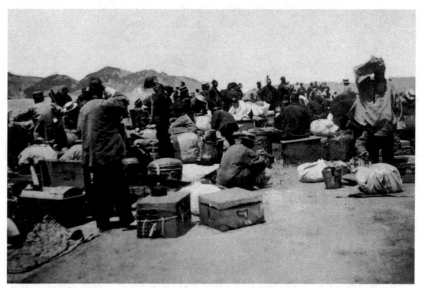

Courtesy NAUS, RG 90, Closing and fastening of suitcases after luggage disinfection, Angel Island, CA.

Fortunately, in 1896, nature again remained within bounds. Of the 196 ships inspected in the Northwest, only 3 vessels were deemed worthy of disinfection. 1,270 passengers were disinfected, regardless of whether they arrived from China, Japan, or anywhere else. 4,709 sailors and 271 pieces of luggage were also inspected.

[55] U.S. Surgeon General Report, report medical Office in Command, Wm G. Stimpson, past assistant. July 29, 1896.

All in all, only 4 patients had to be treated before they proceeded to Seattle or Tacoma and one person was investigated for cholera.

In San Francisco, nine vessels had to be quarantined and disinfected. Their passengers included 1,084 people and were checked in great detail of whom 43 had to be vaccinated and 1,034 bathed, their clothing and baggage were disinfected. In addition, several hundred bags of mail from Asia were opened. That meant that each letter was punctured, spread out, and fumigated. Zero cases of plague had come through!

And yet, in the midst of these scary challenges, commercial traffic only expanded. From San Diego, reports announced "rigidly increasing traffic with China and Japan."Commercial traffic across the Pacific was steadily increasing.

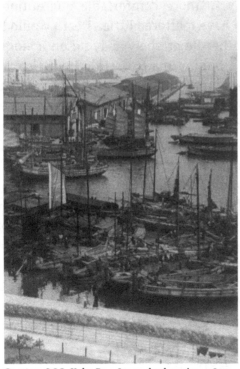

Courtesy LOC, Kobe Bay, Japan, harbor view, 1890.

Most importantly, such expansion was never limited to interaction with China. In San Diego, a large Japanese steamship company expressed interest in acquiring docking privileges. Within 9 months, 4,000 and 5,000-ton steamers were expected to appear on the horizon having crossed from Yokohama to Honolulu to San Diego.[56] It did not take long to ask about distinguishing between infected people arriving in steerage and upper-class people arriving with plague.

Ever since the Middle Ages, the presence of plague had been used as a teaching moment, reminding everybody that disease and death did not distinguish between paupers, peasants, or bishops. Plague was an equal opportunity affair. Yet in 1896 transport lines suggested that Upper-Middle-class plague victims should be locked away in more comfortable quarantine locations. In reality it would have mattered little. Death would have held onto the victim whether he or she was lying on a single bed covered with linen or a bumpy mattress filled with straw. Also, upper crust passengers on their last days on earth would be expected to stand in line on the wharf waiting for inspection, exposed to fog and cold ocean wind like all the rest. Their last bath would also not be anything special. Seagulls screaming would flow over poor and rich passengers alike.[57]

But we should not remain focused exclusively on the absence or presence of plague. How complex and non-stereotypical the health situation was in our country becomes apparent as we examine the 1896 statistics. Even though the U.S.M.H.S. tried to keep smallpox from coming into the country, in 1896, the disease inside the U.S. remained present in 22 states and 74 county and municipal districts. Louisiana had the most cases but a visitor could also catch smallpox in Arkansas, Ohio, Wisconsin or Illinois.

[56] U.S. Surgeon General report 1895, p. 545.
[57] U.S. Surgeon General, Report, p. 554.

New York and Pennsylvania reported 13 cases. In China, plague used the Yangtze River to advance to the ocean and along the coastline. In the U.S., the Mississippi likewise allowed smallpox to slip into the Midwest.

Suddenly, in mid–January, 1897, the effort to obtain money for a station in Astoria revived in the U.S. Congress. On January 16, 1897, the initiative was scheduled to be read in March.[58] Indeed, on March 19, the bill was read twice and again referred to the Committee on Commerce. Four days later, on March 23 , Senator McBride introduced the bill S. 1142.[59]

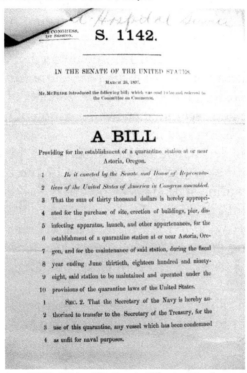

Courtesy NAUS, RG 90, U.S. Senate Bill 1142, March 23, 1897.

[58] NAUS, RG 90, Central File, 1897-1923, Supervising Surgeon General to J.H. Mitchell, U.S. Senate, March 7 1896.
[59] NAUS, RG 90, Central File, 1897-1923, S1142, in the Senate. Providing for the establishment, March 23rd, 1897.

The 1897 proceedings brought some important definitions. For the first time, a written record mentioned a specific location for a future station. It was supposed to be located in the state of Washington, "across the river from Astoria in Pacific County." Specifically, it named "a tract of land north of and adjacent to Knappton Cove's property." Many other locations were ruled out because people lived too close to a hospital where infected individuals would potentially have to spend time. Other locations endangered arriving ships with bad currents.

In March 1898, the Secretary of the Treasury sent S.966 to the House. In April, the Senate discussed the bill again, with updates from the Senate proceedings. The Committee on Interstate and Foreign Commerce, presented by a Mr. Corliss, stated that 1. "in the interest of commerce" and, 2.) "the protection of the health of the people from the invasion of pestilential disease,"[60] the Secretary of Treasury and the Surgeon General of the Marine Hospital Service had recommended the creation of a station and the amount of $30,000 was mentioned.[61]

Three years of legislative effort finally came to a successful end. On May 18, 1897, the 55th Congress of the U.S. provided funds for a quarantine station at the mouth of the Columbia. The U.S. Senate and the House of Representatives endorsed today's equivalent of $840,000 to fund the process of creating a station between 1896 and 1897. The money was to pay for locating land, starting a title search, and assembling buildings: a wharf, a hospital and auxiliary buildings.[62]

On the long journey to making the station a reality, the stretch dedicated to obtaining federal funding had at last been accomplished. Next came finding a location, building the facility, and opening it.

[60] NAUS, RG 90, Central File, 1897–1923, March 3, 1898, Report No. 626 to accompany S 966, House of Representatives.
[61] NAUS, RG 90, Central File, 1897–1923, S 966 An Act.
[62] Ibid., Win R. Cox Secretary, S 966, An Act Providing for the establishment of a quarantine station.

Courtesy NAUS, U.S. Senate Bill 906, accompanying report March 3rd, 1898.

§§§

It had taken four years, from 1894 until 1898, to convince Congress to finance a station on the Columbia River. Finding a location, securing it, and preparing a building would take only four months.

On August 18, 1898, the Treasury Department ordered the assembling of a board tasked with finding an appropriate location. Three stakeholders were represented. The team would consist, first, of William F. Kilgore from the U.S. Revenue Cutter Service steamer "Perry" stationed at Astoria. The second member, by coincidence, was D.A. Carmichael who was on his way to assume office at the U.S. quarantine facilities in Honolulu. He was asked to travel through Astoria to represent the interests of the U.S. Marine Hospital Service.

The third person was John Fox.[63] In the best American tradition, he represented more than one interest. Having originally come to Astoria from British Canada, for years, he had successfully represented the U.S. Customs Service, holding office at the first official customs house west of the Mississippi. A replica stands in Astoria's east end today, near the Safeway supermarket.

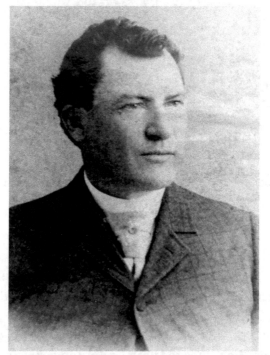

Courtesy Clatsop County Historical Society, John Fox, Astoria, Oregon.

[63] U.S. Department of Health, Annual Report 1897-1898, 740-741.

Fox earned income from supplying the canning industry up and down the West Coast. Just as in San Francisco, where store owners had sold Levis jeans and shovels to miners during the California Gold Rush and found prosperity, Fox invented and manufactured canning machinery. Fox was a major regional entrepreneur who tinkered with the industrial process of making canning easier and cheaper. On and off, new patents attracted merchants all the way from Europe to Astoria. Close to where Pig 'N Pancake today beckons tourists for a delicious breakfast, these merchants checked in at Fox's company office.

The U.S. Treasury Department brought the three men together and asked them to select a location. They were part of an open political process. It invited interested citizens to come to the one federal building in Astoria that symbolized the aspirations of the U.S. government in Oregon and Astoria. The federal tax collection office and the U.S. post office were located there.

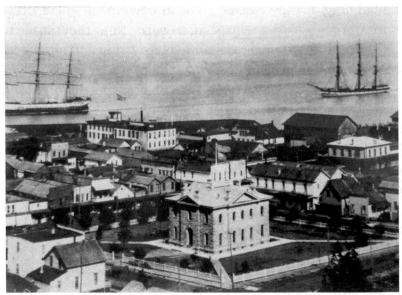

Courtesy Clatsop County Historical Society, Place of decision making: old Office of Customs and Post Office.

On September 1, 1898, at 10 a.m., the three men opened the governmental bidding process in western Astoria at the Custom and Post Office Building between 7th and 8th street. Thereafter ,the group would tour potential sites and return to the federal building for a short period for public comment.[64]

Carmichael, Fox, and Kilgore seemed to have open minds about where a potential quarantine station could be located, but the sources do not tell us of discussions about specific locations in town or the business community's preference.

It was logical to establish quarantine stations where people were suffering from most infectious diseases far outside the city. There, they would be less likely to transmit those diseases to others. Still, officials in Washington, D.C., imagined an "Astorian station."

They had no intention of distinguishing between Oregon and Washington as far as the future siting of a station was concerned. One building already existed right in downtown where Oregon doctors organized their inspection work. Now they needed to find a second, additional location to place a ship and hundreds of people, should they be in need of healing for four weeks.

The three men walked the three blocks north to Astoria's downtown waterfront, boarded the S.S. *Perry*, and floated to the first potential location. In reality, there was little need to do so since, once again, nature was to determine the outcome but in addition, most land on both sides of the river had already been sold and was unavailable. The sources do not say that the group, in theory, ever contemplated claiming "public domain." Finding land certainly meant picking a ground or site that was available

[64] NAUS, RG 90, Central File, 1897-1923, Howell, Washington, Office of the Secretary, Treasury Department Assistant Secretary to Captain W.F. Kilgore, Comd. U.S. Steamer *Perry*, Astoria Oregon, August 18, 1898. Ibid., W.B. Assistant Secretary W.B. Howell to W.F. Kilgore, Commanding U.S. Steamer *Perry*. Astoria Oregon, August 18, 1898. On August 18, Assistant Secretary of Treasury, wrote to Captain W.F. Kilgore that he was supposed to provide services to the newly appointed team

according to U.S. law. In 1898, most prime locations with accessible shoreline were in the hands of former homesteaders or speculators waiting for the railroad boom that so infuriatingly refused to materialize.

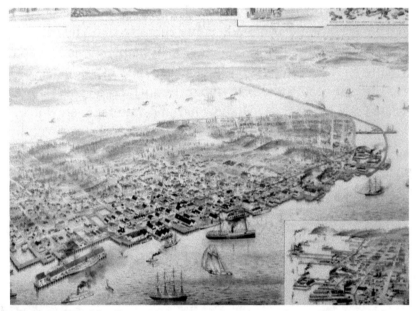

Courtesy Astoria Public Library, Most of the territory the search committee explored, map, Astoria and surroundings, 1898.

The decisive factor, however, was the need to find a place where a ship could find calm rest and not run aground. Ships needed enough water under their keel to cut safely through the bay to the wharf at the station. In addition, the ship needed to be brought close enough to the coast so that ill individuals could be physically transported on stretchers to a yet-to-be built hospital building. Lastly, the anchor needed to allow permanent stationing and easy coming and going, unencumbered by low and high tides. This had nothing to do with being pro-Oregon or pro-Washington. The question was only about geography, about respecting the space that nature had carved out under the bay's surface.

The three men visited southern locations first which were quickly ruled out due to the narrowness of the existing channels. Locations up the river to the east were surveyed next but here too, only limited anchorage existed. Likewise, the areas between Fort Stevens and Astoria were declared off limits, because too large a population was already living there so that any escape of a virus would immediately endanger healthy population clusters.

Above ground, Young's Bay looked vast and was considered to have some desirable features. Under the surface, however, nature revealed a comparatively shallow bar and waters. Even worse, it could be reached only by passing under a drawbridge. Young's Bay was out. Next, the three visited Sand Island. There it became apparent that shifting sand, the island's constant exposure to the sea, and the unsafe anchorage in the vicinity made it undesirable as well. Thereafter, the S.S. *Perry* skirted to the North Shore as far as Knappton Salmon Cannery.

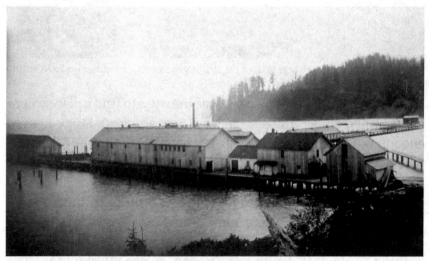

Courtesy Nancy and Rex Anderson and the Bell family, The cannery ready to be converted into a quarantine station.

There, the group left the ship and climbed onto a cannery wharf that welcomed them 50 feet from the shallow sloped shore. They thoroughly examined the property. Here, the Board found a plant of some size. It had recently been a fish canning station, and was located in a beautiful cove as shown on the chart just above Cliff Point. It had four large buildings in fair condition, which, at reasonable expense, could be made serviceable for a quarantine station for storage, disinfecting purposes, barracks for detaining passengers, and so on.[65]

Almost best of all, this land located right at the edge of water, was for sale by its owner. While not excellent, the building's state was in fair repair. The largest building measured 600 by 200 feet. Still, it was not an ideal place:

> Considerable part of the piling is gone above low water mark, but with reasonable expense could be put in good condition. Below low water mark it lasts for years, as the teredo does not exist in these waters, and repairs can be made by cutting off the old piling and setting new timbers upon them which is the usual custom of repairing wharfs in these waters.

Item after item offered possibilities. Even at low tide, there was about 20 feet of water, under a ship's keel at the end of the wharf, but the wharf could be readily extended to deeper water if deemed necessary. The rise and fall of the tide in this locality was about 8 feet so the water's depth was sufficient to accommodate ocean-going vessels. In addition, it offered anchorage without having to deal with shifting sands. They noted that "the area of this cove is some 25 or 30 acres and convenient and safe anchorage for large vessels lies close at hand." Across the bay Astoria could be seen about six miles away.

[65] Ibid.

65

The team quickly envisioned building "a small hospital" without adjacent grounds offering specifics. The group also noticed natural attributes that would help to run a small hospital:

> A desirable feature of this site is a bountiful supply of fine mountain stream water, already on the ground and carried by piping to the end of the wharf. The supply is abundant for all possible needs. The soil is high, dry, and gravelly and some parts are under cultivation. Fine shade and fruit trees also increase the desirability of this location.

There, a quarantine station could open sooner rather than later. Several dwellings already existed on the property, which, as Fox wrote, could be readily converted into quarters for attendants or other purposes. A sawmill was conveniently located about a mile from the cove.

After studying the cannery site, however, the three men did not stop exploring other locations. Four other places were visited, including property belonging to a Mr. McGowan. But, in the end, nowhere did they find conditions as advantageous as those at Knappton Cove. They concluded:

> No other places presented advantages, equal to or in any way approaching those set forth above. The anchorages are more exposed, tides are stronger, and costs of improvements would be very much greater.

It was still early in the evening, around 6:30 p.m., when the S.S. *Perry* crossed the Columbia back to Astoria. On the evening of the same day, September 1, the three men agreed that Knappton Cove should be proposed to the U.S. Treasury administrators awaiting the official suggestion in Washington, D.C. They reported:

it is the opinion of the board after a careful consideration of all points that the location of the Quarantine Station at Knappton Washington, in case the property can be purchased will be to the best interests of the government.

Fox, the local voice, painted a scenario where the existing buildings could be converted to serve health-related functions with relative ease. His assessment was that of a person used to making quick, independent decisions in private business. In theory, a cannery processing plant could be turned into a quarantine station. In reality, however, as part of a bureaucratic process, accounting for every demolition and replacement and hosting subsequent public biddings takes a lot of time. Finding an empty space and building a station from scratch would have been faster, easier, and more appropriate, given the approaching health crisis. The group had not picked a spot that would make it possible to hit the ground running to engage plague head on.

Opportunities for the public to comment were minimal. Perhaps giving 12 hours notice was normal in Astoria, but it also made sure that most local people could not attend on such short notice to object to the board's selection. But such as it was, they offered the opportunity on September 2, 1898, at 2 pm, on the second floor of the Customs house and Post Office.

The sources give no idea whether this process was a contested one or whether those with power in the city were eager to conclude quickly and successfully. Most probably desired was to have a station, any station, plus a regular budget from Washington, D.C. After all, it had taken four years of legislative committee work to receive this appropriation. Not spending the money during the assigned budget cycle would have amounted to a declaration of political bankruptcy by local politicians, their representatives in Congress, and commercial circles.

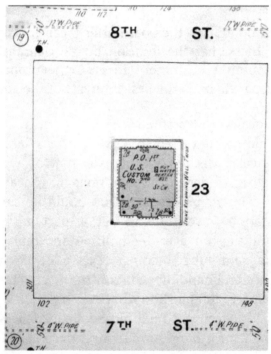

Courtesy Clatsop County Historical Society, Excerpt from insurance map: drawing of Astoria's Custom House and Post Office.

Still, one public comment appears in the record. A Dr. A.C. Kinney advocated placing the station on the south side of the Columbia along Young's River. This was an interjection by a health professional who failed to realize that nature offered limited options. Below the river's surface lurked shoalwater approaches unsuitable for larger ships. After a few minutes of discussion, Dr. Kinney withdrew his objection.

Nobody from the Washington side of the river seemed to have crossed the bay to come to the customs house and post office to participate in the hearing. Even though the quarantine station was to be on the Washington side, no person living there filed an objection.

In addition to finding a geographical location for the station, another question concerned where to put the infected ballast from ships. Today, one would expect such an issue to create a heated discussion and much popular antipathy to having a potentially dangerous station nearby. Yet the record of the discussions on September 2 reports that the discussion was merely postponed for a later time.

The two meetings seemed to have been a well-managed public process leading as fast as possible to spending the federal money for the desired station. After only one hour, the public hearing was adjourned. Astorian politicians and commercial and shipping interests had moved closer to having their station.

Two weeks later, Treasury Department bureaucrats from Washington, D.C. asked for an update. So, on October 3, John Fox, accompanied by an unknown man, took a boat and again crossed the river to inspect the Knappton cannery property for a second time.

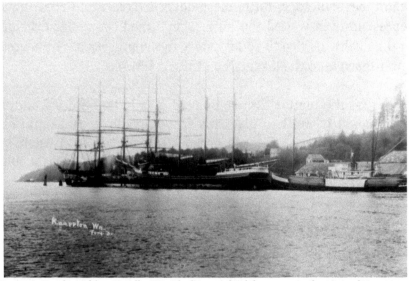

Courtesy Appelo Archive, Naselle, WA; The bay south of the cannery: the town of Knappton and her mill.

This time he focused his interest on the specifics of the buildings. He reported that the main cannery building was 400 x 50 feet long with a depth of 200 feet. The property included a main dwelling house, five small cottages, and minor buildings. The cannery supervisor's house had 2.5 stories, 12 rooms, closets, pantries, and large woodsheds.[66]

At that point, the selection committee declared its task accomplished. The search had produced a viable location. Local business and shipping interests as well as local doctors, accepted the cannery site as "most suitable."[67]

If these men had their way and the Treasury Department followed their suggestion a land and water location had been found that could become, over the years, a building where federal quarantine station procedures could take place although it would require major rebuilding and much investment.

However, Astorians pressured decision makers in the nation's capital not to drop the ball. The group wrote that the cannery might be sold to a different bidder if Treasury Department representatives waited too long. They urged the upper echelon of the health service to add its voice to the process. One undated letter insisted to the leadership of the U.S.M.H.S.

> that the matter cannot be held openly indefinitely and it would be well to give this fact immediate consideration as they have business prospects that may lead them to withdraw their proposal if not accepted within a reasonable time.[68]

---

[66] NAUS, RG 90, Central File, 1897-1923, Letter to Secretary of Treasury, October 3, 1898. The second page of this letter is missing. The source fails to realize that the house was the house of Cannery Superintendent. Joseph Hume never lived in this house.
[67] NAUS, RG 90, Central File, 1897-1923, Letter to Secretary of the Treasury, Office of the Collector of Customs, Fox, October 3, 1898.
[68] NAUS, RG 90, Central File, 1897-1923, signed by Fox, Captain Kilgore, and Carmichael.

The historical record does not suggest any hint that a rival bidder was competing or waiting in the wings. To the contrary, Astoria's cannery boom fever of earlier years had ended. Perhaps owner Hume was even glad to have found a buyer.

The bureaucrats in the Treasury Department refused to be pressured. As in any modern real estate deal, a survey of the land had to be made plus a title search. Even so, the men on the East Coast had already accepted the Northwest's selection and assumed that the searches turned up only good news. No one suggested moving the searches to the Oregon side or building a station from scratch.

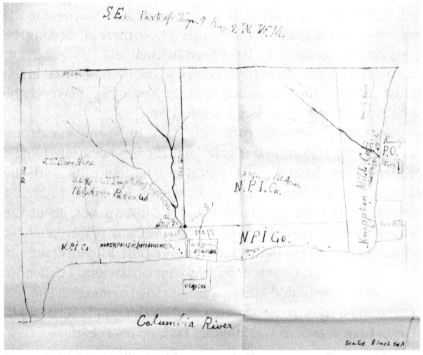

Courtesy NAUS, RG 90, Earliest hand drawn map of wider area surrounding quarantine station property, around 1900.

A few days after Thanksgiving, 1898, with the rainy season approaching, on November 29, a Secretary of the Treasury's representative ordered an official survey of the cannery's entire territory and property. The Treasury offered also $35 dollars to pay Captain Kilgore to conduct the survey.

After taking the S.S. *Perry* across the river, Kilgore encountered another Washingtonian, a Mr. Callender, the owner of the adjacent property adjacent to the east. He was a prominent figure in Knappton and also served as president of a real estate investment company called the North Pacific Improvement Company. As the company's president he was tied to an investment office in Spokane Washington. The investors had paid $800 dollars per acre. What would the presence of a quarantine station next to the property do for the value of the property? Even more interesting the president on the national level lived in Litchfield,[69] Connecticut. Callender's opposition to the station had not been reported in the initial report from September 1898. In November, however, he sought to defeat the cannery's acquisition.

Kilgore had actually come not just to examine existing property, but also to investigate land further north of Hume's cannery. Even that early, the parcel of land that came with the existing cannery buildings was considered too small to host a modern station. When Kilgore asked for information about the price of the five acres north and west of the cannery lot, Callender refused to provide the figure. Later in his report, Kilgore described the exchange with Callender as "very unsatisfactory." Callender did more than withhold information. He tried to make an end run around supporters in Astoria. He asked Washington's Senator J.C. Wilson to intervene in Washington, D.C., on his behalf.[70]

---

[69] In 1916 Mr. G.S. McNeill in Litchfield, Connecticut was listed as president of the North Pacific Improvement Co. NAUS, RG 90, North Pacific Improvement Co. to R.H.Creel, Assistant Surgeon General.
[70] NAUS, RG 90, Central File, 1897–1923, Letter, Fox to Secretary of State, December 17, 1898.

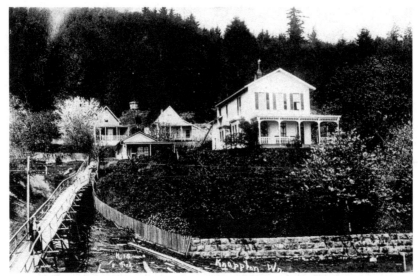

Courtesy Appelo Archives, Naselle, WA, City block in Knappton where Mr. Callender's house was located.

Back in Astoria, Kilgore simply continued finishing the application package. Maps were prepared and descriptions written and then they were sent, mailed by train or ship to Washington, D.C. The selection committee had accomplished all its necessary work in 4 months as it informed the federal government on December 17, 1898.[71]

In theory, the sale of the cannery to the Department of Treasury might still collapse for some unlikely reason. The Hume brothers had not yet received payment nor had the deed been recorded therefore the sale could technically still be voided.

Moreover, Callender continued to fight. Five days after the Astorian committee mailed the documentation off to Washington, D.C., Callender wrote to Senator Wilson there. Thus, on December 22, he asked the senator to do what was possible to "prevent gross injustice."

[71] NAUS, RG 90, Central File, 1897-1923, Letter, John Fox Collector of Customs and member of board to Secretary of Treasury, December 17, 1898. Voucher for services of Mrs. Tee and Bell, Surveyors in amount of 35 $ dollars. Here with payment recommended

Friedrich E. Schuler

Courtesy NAUS, RG 90, Letter, M.P. Callender to Senator Hon. John L. Wilson, December 22, 1898.

In contrast to the selection committee, he described a far less harmonious true process that had led to the selection of the cannery site. He claimed that Astorian citizens had engaged in persistent petitioning to obtain federal money to secure a station for the bay. But he thought that the selection did not offer a predictable safe path for ships to reach their place to anchor.

74

Instead, they had picked Knappton to push dangerous pathogens out of their town. They were met at every turn with resistance by Oregon residents. Thus, they were compelled to go and look on the other side of the sound on the coast of Washington, he argued. There a piece of land was owned by somebody with ties to Astoria. He promised a reasonable price. Now it had been selected against the wishes and protests of Mr. Callender and the North Pacific Improvement Company.

Callender, like many others, seemed oblivious to the very real danger of an epidemic infecting citizens in the Northwest. He saw the land next to Hume's cannery narrowly only as an object of railroad land speculation. He, the company, and investors outside Oregon had invested $4,201,600[72] to build Knappton, the mill, wharfs and warehouses.

He considered it disagreeable to place a quarantine station next to what he was building and an injustice to the company's business interests. Now that the quarantine station might be put in the very heart of his piece of land it "will utterly disvalue the capital invested there." He therefore asked decision makers in Washington, D.C., to see the station's placement as a highly partisan Oregonian deal against the interest of people on the Washington side. He predicted that, given time, all Washingtonians would oppose this station opening at Hume's cannery site.[73]

But Callender and his investors failed to find even a single active sympathetic supporter in the nation's capital. By December 30, John Fox knew that the U.S. government had accepted the proposed site formerly occupied by the Eureka Company. Only the title remained to be examined and approved.[74]

[72] This is the 2014 inflation adjusted value of $150,000. Calculated through web egg.com 2/8/2015.
[73] NAUS, RG 90 , Central File, 1897–1923, Letter, Mr. Callender to U.S. Senator John L. Wilson, U.S. Senator, December 22, 1898.
[74] NAUS, RG 90, Central File, 1897–1923, Eureka and Epicure Morning Co. to John Fox, Collector of Customs, Astoria, Ore. January 30th, 1899.

The new year, 1899, began with cannery owner Hume's urgent inquiry about when his company would receive payment from the federal government. On January 30, 1899, the cannery owners wrote to Fox that they were ready to transfer the property and asked to confirm the result of the title search. If examiners in D.C. or Oregon had any questions left, the cannery would be glad to make available the complete abstract of this property if they were asked to do so.[75]

This nudge brought no closure. A second nudge came from Congress when the Committee on Coast Defenses inquired about the status of the acquisition process. They insisted that the business community in Astoria was on pins and needles to have the deal signed for good:

> permit me to say that business men of Astoria and of Portland and owners of steamship lines doing business between Columbia River and Oriental ports are exceedingly anxious of the early construction of the quarantine station, realizing as they do that the necessity for its use may become almost imperative any week or any month.[76]

Even though the Treasury Department had held out the possibility of payment within two to three months, no money had been paid by June 1899. Perhaps 1899 commercial culture was such that it mattered less. In any case, by May, the U.S. Marine Hospital Service officially established its federal presence in the heart of Oregon's health service, with all the powers that came with it.

In the second week of May 1899, George Hill Hastings, reported for duty as the first federal station master. In 1897, he

[75] NAUS, RG 90, Central File, 1897-1923, Eureka and Epicure Morning Co. to John Fox, Collector of Customs, Astoria, Ore. January 30th, 1899.
[76] NAUS, RG 90, Central File, 1897-1923, Committee on Coast Defenses, U.S. Senate, Geowwer Bride to Walter Wyman, SSG, February 3rd 1899.

served at New Orleans' station. In early 1898, he had filled in Middleborough, Kentucky. Now he worked at the mouth of the Columbia River. He was to lead a life of service, serving two regions, one on each side of the Columbia River. In Oregon, his medical office would continue to be located in downtown Astoria. In Washington State, at the cannery building six miles across from Astoria, he was to realize the conversion of the cannery into a quarantine station where ships could be fumigated safely and ill passengers quarantined.

After one month of work however, he too faced Hume's anger about still not having been paid. On July 11, they requested "immediate payment, desirous to have the matter closed up."[77]

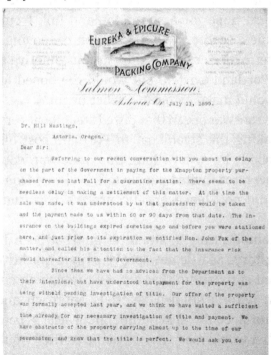

Courtesy NAUS, RG 90, "Where is the money?" letter, cannery owners to U.M.S.

[77] NAUS, RG 90, Central File, 1897-1923, Eureka and Epicure, Letter, President to Hill Hastings, July 11, 1899.

Unfortunately, the records do not allow us to pinpoint the day when finally money was deposited. And thus federal health inspection work of incoming ships was added to Oregon's health service.

When Assistant Surgeon George Hill Hastings arrived in Astoria, he found the context for his work in a state of continuous and expanding change. He assumed his post on April 28, 1899.[78]

A few weeks earlier, the railroad gap between Gobel and Astoria had been closed. On April 3, the last spike was hammered into the ground next to the Columbia. On April 11, Astoria's subsidy committee rode over the new tracks to Goble and returned to Astoria the same day. Afterward, they voted the contract fulfilled. The theoretical hope for a shore-to-land link from Asia could finally become a reality. Now, the option of moving freight and people by sternwheeler, steamship, and locomotive between the Pacific and Portland existed. But would the hoped for economic boom that would make Astorians richer begin?

No, only a rate war began that pitted steamboat versus railroad. Suddenly, taking the steamboat to Portland cost only 25 cents one way. Nobody knew how long this price war would last. The incredible low fares invited people to travel east from September 1899 on. It did not, however, encourage a trip from Astoria to Asia.

Further complicating the situation, gold had been discovered in Alaska's territory. Seattle newspaper writers quickly whipped up an unjustified enthusiasm that echoed through an entire nation. Dreamers in Astoria studied Seattle's approach and pondered whether Astoria could also jump on Seattle's bandwagon or imitate it. That would mean that "Pacific traffic" would no longer be comprised of traffic from Astoria to Asia, but also from Astoria

[78] I am grateful to retired U.S.M.H.S. officer Jay Paulsen, Hillsboro, Oregon, for sharing with me the data he collected detailing the career of the surgeons. For additional information see his link at the Knappton Cove Heritage Museum online exhibit.

to Seattle and Alaska. As early as 1897, this potential already intoxicated speculators in Astoria when the ship *Elder* stopped in port.[79]

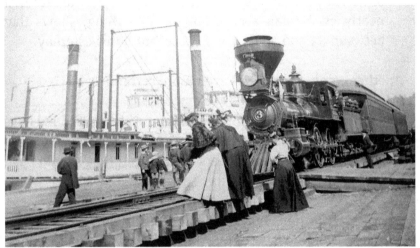

Courtesy Clatsop County Historical Society, *The Railroad has arrived in Astoria!*

The *Elder* transported 400 prospectors into town. More importantly, it carried on board $5,602,187 in cash and $5,600,000 in supplies, according to a conservative estimate.[80] One writer captured the excitement and hope for increased traffic in the Astoria newspaper:

> the busy scene enacted at the locks yesterday and the life on the streets was a realistic picture of what Astoria will be when the loading of an ocean steamer is a daily occurrence and a trade is established with Alaska, Japan, China, and other countries. All day the merchants were as busy as they could be supplying the last wants of the passengers of the Elder destined to the land of wealth at the far north.

[79] Newspaper article Astoria Oregon Sunday Morning, August 1, 1897.
[80] Based on inflation currency converter for the year 1897. Calculated on February 7, 2015 at westegg.com

Nearly everyone had forgotten several articles necessary to their comfort and took advantage of the delay of the ship to purchase in Astoria. A careful estimate made on the basis of actual purchases by a dozen or more, and the fact that nearly every man aboard bought something, shows that between $3,500 and $4,000 was spent here yesterday.

Another commentator was even more certain:

Alaska business has come to stay. Astoria and Portland have been slow in grasping the situation, but with one steamer in the line to stay and others in prospect, they should push trade with that territory day and night.[81]

At the same time, but not connected, political groups in Washington D.C. who favored U.S. imperialism abroad, made their wishes known to the president in the White House in several ways. By June, 1898, Hawaii was no longer an independent kingdom but an annexed territory of the United States. More significantly, the 1898 war with Spain's world empire had begun.[82] In April 1898, President William McKinley finally gave in to popular pressure and launched the U.S. war against Spain. Oregon volunteers formed the 2nd Oregon Volunteer infantry and traveled to the Philippine islands. The Oregonians stopped in Honolulu on June 1 and arrived in Manila Bay on June 30, 1898. They besieged the Spanish troops there and captured Manila on August 13, 1898.

[81] *Astoria Herald*, August 14, 1897. Some wealthy Astorians were mad with dreams about profiting from the news of Klondike's bonanza. They wanted to build a dozen steamboats for the Alaska trade at a supposed cost of $ 2,000,000 Alaska and Steamboat Company. "The object of the company will be to grubstake anybody who wants to go to Alaska."
[82] In August 14, 1897 among the most active workers and faithful attendants of the Chamber of Commerce were Judge Gray, Judge Bowlby, James W. Welch G Wingate and E. C. Holden. These people were considered old timers and they considered many projects that turned out not to be lucrative. September 12, 1897.

The region was full of yellow fever and other dangerous diseases that had not yet been introduced into the U.S. Northwest. It was not clear when the soldiers would return home but, as of 1898, no building or location existed in Astoria that would offer a place for Oregon volunteers to recover upon their return.

Radically, commercial transport to the Northwest increased. A look at the number of ships arriving in Puget Sound reveals within 12 months the number of ships had nearly doubled from 196 to 370 vessels. Inspectors requested 11,271 sailors and 4,796 passengers to walk by them. Of these, 438 were detained and 801 pieces of luggage spent a night next to the sulfur pots. Such vigilance paid off. Only two smallpox cases were found and both of the men survived.[83]

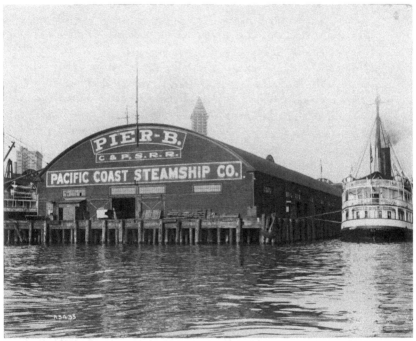

Courtesy Seattle MOIA, 1978.6585.4atif, Seattle Dock of Pacific Coast Steamship Co.

[83] U.S. Surgeon General Annual Report, 1896–1897, p. 507.

In Astoria, companies now openly joined the efforts of the health service and Oregon politicians. In July, 1898, a company's letterhead appeared in the surviving sources for the first time. On July 2, 1898, the Dodwell and Carlill Company office from Portland wrote to Surgeon General Walter Wyman in Washington, D.C.

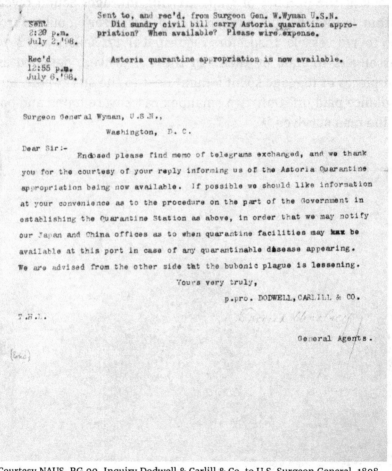

Courtesy NAUS, RG 90, Inquiry Dodwell & Carlill & Co. to U.S. Surgeon General, 1898.

In 1891, its original office had opened in San Francisco and by 1898, it maintained branches in Portland, Tacoma, and Victoria B.C.[84] Representing the North Pacific Steamship Company,[85] the company was aware that bill S.966 had been negotiated and its representative wanted to know the outcome: "in order that we may notify our Japan and China offices as to when quarantine facilities may be available at this port in case of any quarantinable disease appearing." They insisted there was no time to allow the answer to reach Portland by mail, instead, it should be telegraphed at company expense.[86] Four days later, the Washington office of the Surgeon General replied that the Astoria quarantine appropriation had been approved.

On July 18, the Astoria Chamber of Commerce seconded the Portland company's push to speed matters up. Astorian business representatives also wanted "work to be expedited as much as is practicable.[87] An unknown senator added pressure on the Senate when he wrote in the same week: "I have no doubt the matter will have your earnest attention as I trust the work will be pushed forward as rapidly as possible."[88]

Once Dodwell & Carlill learned that money had at last been set aside, it took only days to follow up with a request for a detailed timetable of when construction could be expected to take place.[89] Two days later, Dodwell & Carlille repeated their request.

[84] B. Olney Hough, *American Exporter's Export Trade Directory*, (New York: American Exporter Johnston, Export Publisher, 1919.) 6th edit, p. 285. In 1920 it was listed as importer and exporter of general machinery, iron and steel products, electrical and railway materials, machine tools, hardware chemicals, California canned fruits, sardines, and all American manufacturer and grown products.

[85] It was founded on March 7, 1869. It purchased the property and shares of the California, Oregon and Mexican Steamship Company. New York Times, March 7, 1869 p. 5.

[86] NAUS, RG 90, Central File, 1897-1923, Telegram, Dodwell Carlille and Co. to General Wyman, July 2, 1898. The same letter reported that the seriousness of the bubonic plague in China at that time was lessening.

[87] NAUS, RG 90, Central File, 1897-1923, Geonmer Zinda, U.S. Senate to Walter Wyman July 18, 1898.

[88] NAUS, RG 90, Central File, 1897-1923, Geonmer Zinder to Walter Wyman, Supervising Surgeon General, July 18, 1898.

[89] NAUS, RG 90, Central File, 1897-1923, Dodwell Carlille, Northern Pacific Steamship Co, to Dr. Preston H. Bailhache, July 20, 1898.

This time, they wanted to know the timetable for selecting a commission that could tour the mouth of the Columbia to find the right site and also the timetable for construction. They added further insight into their motivation:

> This office feared that money would be lost for their customers if their ships would have to be sent to Port Townsend. They wanted to avoid great loss of money. Moreover, if efforts would not work out this time, they asked the Navy in Washington, D.C., to devise temporary facilities in case of need. They were hoping that local health officials could inform them.[90]

From June of 1898 on, the U.S. Marine Hospital Service performed its task on the Astoria side of the bay where the agency inspected 44 ships until June 1900. Of these, 16 passed without having to interrupt their journey but 28 had to be quarantined and disinfected.

Fortunately, no dangerous health emergency was encountered while only 5 crews of only 5 ships had to be disinfected. Still, 85% passed without problem. Even so, that still meant looking at 6,120 individuals, most of them crew members, though only two had to be detained temporarily. Their diagnosis was not shared. If they were kept on a ship anchored at Knappton, or in Astoria, the historical record does not state. One had picked up yellow fever during a prior voyage; three cases of beriberi were also registered.

The ships themselves also arrived in an acceptable state of operation. Of the 44 ships, 42 had cabins that were all certified as clean. Only 2 ships had cabins that also housed rats and lice and had to be fumigated. Of 19 ships arriving from Honolulu, 16 had their holds disinfected to destroy rats.

[90] NAUS, RG 90, Central File, 1897–1923, Letter, Northern Pacific Steam Company, Portland Oregon, represented by Dodwell and Carlille and Co. July 20, 1898.

The most important item still to be dealt with was luggage. An astounding 1,526 pieces of luggage were fumigated after standing on Astoria's wharf. Boxes and cargo from 28 ships had to be showered with sulfur vapor because their place of origin had reported the presence of plague.

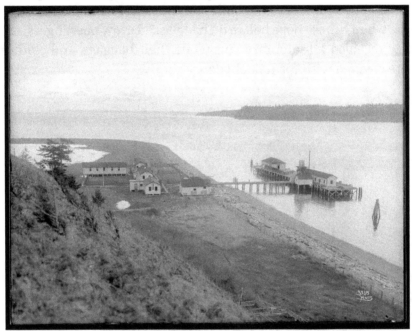

Courtesy Seattle Museum of Science and History, 1983.10.7345.tif, Modernized Quarantine Station Port Townsend.

Eight immigrants arriving from Asia were required to submit their baggage for disinfection.

The brunt of the work continued to be realized by the U.S. Marine Hospital Service team in Port Townsend. There, 297 ships were inspected, 8 times as many as in Astoria. 157 of them were sailing ships with the remaining 140 powered by steam.

In addition, 10,055 crew members walked by inspectors and 5,308 passengers were asked if they had been vaccinated against smallpox. If not, the service gave them a vaccination right on the spot. The majority of these people did not come from China. Only 1,099 had come from China while 431 arrived from Japan. The remaining 3,778 men and women were not from Asia at all.

In Port Townsend, a bath house now offered ten showers for men and two for women. A boiler on the wharf heated water. The time when a mere hose had to do had passed. Now passengers and crew received a temporary suit while their baggage and clothes were cleaned with formaldehyde.

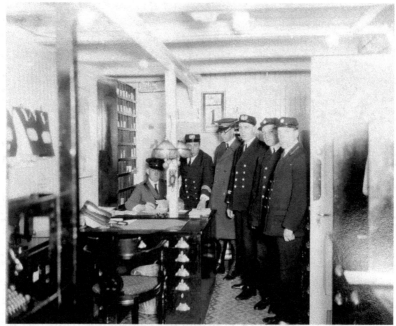

Courtesy NAUS, RG 90, Officers of the U.S.M.H.S., location unknown, no date.

In anticipation of a ship full of infected travelers, a single building was erected to welcome 140 ill passenger or crew. Authorities cut 746 yards of canvas to be made into 165 bunks, a number that would overcrowd the place by 25 should it ever be used.[91]

[91] U.S. Surgeon General Report, 1897-1899, p. 739-740.

Surgeons everywhere were on the lookout for plague, and yet smallpox remained the natural enemy they most often engaged. Every traveler's skin was inspected for signs of a smallpox vaccination and about half had not been vaccinated. Rather than dealing with the illness itself, doctors vaccinated 199 passengers before allowing them to proceed to Tacoma or Seattle.[92]

Suddenly, yellow fever, a most unexpected disease tried to pry its way into the Northwest. Usually, the U.S. Marine Hospital Service had to deal with that deadly disease at stations on the Atlantic side with ships coming from the Caribbean, Panama, or Mexico. In 1899, it wanted to test its mettle in Seattle.

One ship from Panama, the British barque *Cape York*, brought yellow fever to Tacoma. On its deck rested eight people struck down by the fever. Four of them died.[93] That the health service identified the eight people among many thousands of individuals was a major accomplishment.[94] Regular observations continued to examine 7,616 people, 16,672 pieces of luggage, and 57 bags of mail. Each letter was opened and disinfected.

South of Astoria, in San Francisco, Angel Island's lazaretto was also busy. Smooth walls had been installed there to make them easier to scrub or spray after a diseased individual had left traces of the infectious agents dysentery, cholera, and smallpox.[95] Every boat coming from Mexico and further south was carrying passengers ill with yellow fever. Malaria arrived too, and new smallpox cases were introduced from Hong Kong. Now, as a matter of principle, all baggage and containers from Japan and China were being disinfected.[96]

---

[92] U.S. Surgeon General Report, 1897-1898, p.739. Surg. Brook Report P.T. Oct. 5, 1898.
[93] Ibid., 737.
[94] U.S. Surgeon General report 1897-1898, p.739. All in all 15 ships were disinfected. 11 of them had been ships of the passenger liners. 3 were cargo ships and one a bark.
[95] U.S. Surgeon General, Report, 1897-1898, p. 737, Angel Island, M.J Rosenau, p.737.
[96] U.S. Surgeon General Report, 1897-1898, p. 737.

Courtesy NAUS, RG 90; *She exists! Letter with Columbia River Quarantine Station letter head, 1899.*

It was then that the plague finally broke through the second defensive perimeter and appeared in San Francisco's Bay. Three passengers at Angel Island were found to have bubonic swelling, one of them died. This time, the plague remained contained on the island, in viewing distance of San Francisco. It was only a matter of time, however, before it would try again to jump from Honolulu to San Francisco Bay, creep ashore, and move inland.[97]

[97] U.S. Surgeon General Report, 1897-1898, p.737.

In Astoria, individuals of the U.S. Marine Hospital Service finally began to convert the cannery into a quarantine station. Unlike Angel Island or Port Townsend, it was not yet in a position to deal with a major health crisis. It still depended on luck that plague would go elsewhere.

In the previous six years, voices, ideas, plans, and arguments captured on paper had dominated the historical records. Now that a building existed, the next decade would be all about people performing preparatory tasks and doing the specific remodeling to make a cannery into a quarantine station equal to those at Port Townsend and Angel Island. At least, that was the starting point as the new century began.

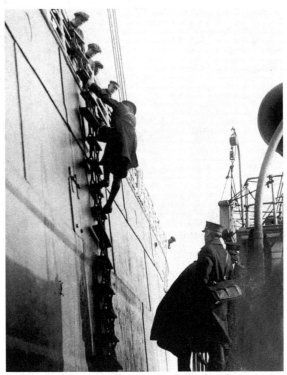

Courtesy NAUS, RG 90, *The inspector climbs aboard.*

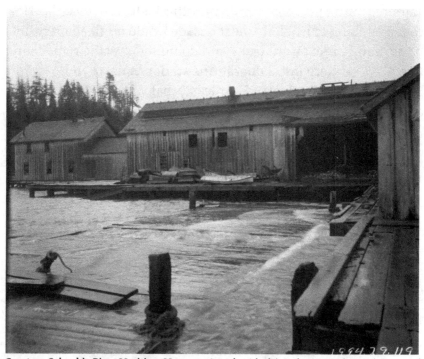

Courtesy Columbia River Maritime Museum, Astoria, *A look into the quarantine station, ground level.*

Bibliography

Primary Sources

National Archives of the United States, Washington, D.C,. RG 90, U.S. Public Health Service.

Astoria Daily Bulletin, **Astoria**.

Astoria Oregon Sunday.

Astoria, Public Library, Records pertaining to the Quarantine Station.

Astoria, Clatsop County Historical Society, Records pertaining to the Quarantine Station.

Knappton Cove Heritage Museum.

California Department of Parks and Recreation, Website.

Pacific Fishermen: Year Book, 1920, based on Columbia Riverimages.com/regions/places. Accessed 2018.

U.S. Surgeon General, The U.S. Surgeon General Report series. U.S. Government Printing Office 1890 to 1900.

San Francisco Call.

Secondary Sources

Books

Anderson, Nancy Bell, Heather Bell Henry, ed.; *The Columbia River's Ellis Island, The Story of Knappton Cove*, **Gearhart: self-published, 2012.**

Mullan, Fitzhugh, M.D., *Plagues and Politis: The Story of the U.S. Public Health Service*, **New York, Basic Books, 1989.**

Markel, Howard, *Quarantine! East European Jewish Immigrants and the New York Epidemics of 1892*, **Baltimore and London: John Hopkins Press, 1997.**

Randall, David K., B*lack Death at Golden Gate: The Race to Save America from the Bubonic Plague*, New York: W. Norton & Co., 2019.

Surgeon General of U.S.P.H.S. and Marine Hospital Service, Washington D.C., Annual Reports, Government Printing Office, Annual Reports, 1877 to 1900.

Online Articles

Becker, Paula, "Federal Maritime Quarantine Station for Puget Sound," History Link.org Essay 8203, James G. Mc Curdy in By Juan de Fuca's Strait, on HistoryLink.org, free online encyclopedia of Washington State History, accessed January 18, 2015.

Lee, Douglas, "Chinese Americans in Oregon." Oregon Encyclopedia.

"Goon Dip," "Moy Bok-Hin," History Link Essay accessed 2016.

"Making History—The Past, Present and Future of the Philadelphia Lazaretto," Oct 19, 2018, accessed March 13, 2020.

"Smallpox Epidemic of 1862 among Northwest Coast and Puget Sound Indians," Washington History Link, encyclopedia.

"The first Salmon Cannery on the Columbia River opens at Eagle Cliff, Wahkiakum Country in 1866 by Kit Oldham," Dec 20, 2006; HistoryLink.org, accessed 2/3/2015.

CPSIA information can be obtained
at www.ICGtesting.com
Printed in the USA
LVHW021649270521
688665LV00021B/1438